MONOGRAPH
IMMUNE-MEDIATED NEUROLOGICAL DISORDERS

MONOGRAPH
IMMUNE-MEDIATED NEUROLOGICAL DISORDERS

Editors

Lakshmi Narasimhan Ranganathan
MD DNB (Internal Medicine) DM (Neuro) DNB (Neuro) PhD (Neuro)
FAAN FRCP (London) FRCP (Glasgow) FACP FIAN MNAMS
Director and Professor of Neurology
Institute of Neurology
Madras Medical College
Chennai, Tamil Nadu, India

Mugundhan Krishnan
MD DM (Neuro) FRCP (Glasgow) FRCP (London)
FRCP (Ireland) FACP (USA) FICP
Professor and Head
Department of Neurology
Government Stanley Medical College
Chennai, Tamil Nadu, India

Rajesh Shankar Iyer
MD DM DNB MNAMS MRCP (UK) (Neurology) FRCP (Glasgow)
Consultant Neurologist and Epileptologist
Kovai Medical Center and Hospitals
Coimbatore, Tamil Nadu, India

Forewords
Rohini Handa
Sudhir V Shah

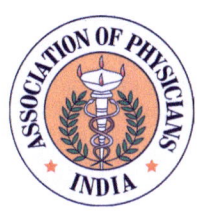

Under the Auspices of Indian College of Physicians,
Academic Wing of the Association of Physicians of India

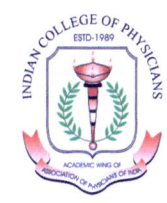

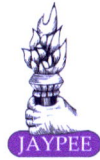

JAYPEE BROTHERS MEDICAL PUBLISHERS
The Health Sciences Publisher
New Delhi | London

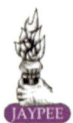 **Jaypee Brothers Medical Publishers (P) Ltd**

Headquarters
EMCA House
23/23-B, Ansari Road, Daryaganj
New Delhi 110 002, India
Landline: +91-11-23272143, +91-11-23272703
+91-11-23282021, +91-11-23245672
E-mail: jaypee@jaypeebrothers.com

Corporate Office
Jaypee Brothers Medical Publishers (P) Ltd.
4838/24, Ansari Road, Daryaganj
New Delhi 110 002, India
Phone: +91-11-43574357
Fax: +91-11-43574314
E-mail: jaypee@jaypeebrothers.com

Overseas Office
JP Medical Ltd.
83, Victoria Street, London
SW1H 0HW (UK)
Phone: +44-20 3170 8910
Fax: +44(0)20 3008 6180
E-mail: info@jpmedpub.com

Website: www.jaypeebrothers.com
Website: www.jaypeedigital.com

© 2022, Indian College of Physicians, Academic Wing of Association of Physicians of India.

The views and opinions expressed in this book are solely those of the original contributor(s)/author(s) and do not necessarily represent those of editor(s) of the book.

All rights reserved by the author. No part of this publication may be reproduced, stored or transmitted in any form or by any means, electronic, mechanical, photocopying, recording or otherwise, without the prior permission in writing of the publishers.

All brand names and product names used in this book are trade names, service marks, trademarks or registered trademarks of their respective owners. The publisher is not associated with any product or vendor mentioned in this book.

Medical knowledge and practice change constantly. This book is designed to provide accurate, authoritative information about the subject matter in question. However, readers are advised to check the most current information available on procedures included and check information from the manufacturer of each product to be administered, to verify the recommended dose, formula, method and duration of administration, adverse effects and contraindications. It is the responsibility of the practitioner to take all appropriate safety precautions. Neither the publisher nor the author(s)/editor(s) assume any liability for any injury and/or damage to persons or property arising from or related to use of material in this book.

This book is sold on the understanding that the publisher is not engaged in providing professional medical services. If such advice or services are required, the services of a competent medical professional should be sought.

Every effort has been made where necessary to contact holders of copyright to obtain permission to reproduce copyright material. If any have been inadvertently overlooked, the publisher will be pleased to make the necessary arrangements at the first opportunity. The **CD/DVD-ROM** (if any) provided in the sealed envelope with this book is complimentary and free of cost. **It is Not meant for sale.**

Inquiries for bulk sales may be solicited at: jaypee@jaypeebrothers.com

Monograph: Immune-mediated Neurological Disorders / Lakshmi Narasimhan Ranganathan, Mugundhan Krishnan, Rajesh Shankar Iyer

First Edition: **2022**

ISBN: 978-93-5270-451-4

Printed in India

Contributors

Editors

Lakshmi Narasimhan Ranganathan MD DNB (Internal Medicine) DM (Neuro) DNB (Neuro) PhD (Neuro) FAAN FRCP (London) FRCP (Glasgow) FACP FIAN MNAMS
Director and Professor of Neurology
Institute of Neurology
Madras Medical College
Chennai, Tamil Nadu, India

Mugundhan Krishnan MD DM (Neuro) FRCP (Glasgow) FRCP (London) FRCP (Ireland) FACP (USA) FICP
Professor and Head
Department of Neurology
Government Stanley Medical College
Chennai, Tamil Nadu, India

Rajesh Shankar Iyer MD DM DNB MNAMS MRCP (UK) (Neurology) FRCP (Glasgow)
Consultant Neurologist and Epileptologist
Kovai Medical Center and Hospitals
Coimbatore, Tamil Nadu, India

Contributing Authors

Afshan Jabeen Shaik DM
Additional Professor of Neurology
Department of Neurology
Nizam's Institute of Medical Sciences
Hyderabad, Telangana, India

Annamma Mathai MSc PhD
Research Scientist
Neuroimmunology Laboratory
Department of Neurology
Amrita Institute of Medical Sciences
Ponekkara Kochi, Kerala, India

Arun Shivaraman Mulanur Murugesan MD
Resident
Institute of Neurology
Madras Medical College
Chennai, Tamil Nadu, India

Balasubramanian Samivel MBBS MD DM
Professor of Neurology
Institute of Neurology
Madras Medical College
Chennai, Tamil Nadu, India

Chandramouleeswaran V MBBS MD DM
Professor of Neurology
Institute of Neurology
Madras Medical College
Chennai, Tamil Nadu, India

Davidson Devasia MD
Senior Resident
Department of Neurology
Amrita Institute of Medical Sciences
Ponekkara, Kochi, Kerala, India

Ganesh Veeraraghavan MBBS MD
Resident
Institute of Neurology
Madras Medical College
Chennai, Tamil Nadu, India

Guhan Ramamurthy MD
Resident
Institute of Neurology
Madras Medical College
Chennai, Tamil Nadu, India

Harish Jayakumar MBBS MD MRCP(UK) DM
Neurologist
JK Institute of Neurology
Madurai, Tamil Nadu, India

Jawahar Marimuthu MBBS MD DM
Professor of Neurology
Institute of Neurology
Madras Medical College
Chennai, Tamil Nadu, India

Kalpana D MD DM DNB
Consultant Pediatric Neurologist
Kerala Institute of Medical Sciences (KIMS) Hospital
Thiruvananthapuram, Kerala, India

Kannan Vangiliappan MD DM
Consultant Neurologist
Purnalakshmi Neuro Centre
Karimnagar, Telangana, India

Kaushik MG MBBS MD DM
Consultant Neurologist
Sri Ramakrishna Hospital
Coimbatore, Tamil Nadu, India

Krishnamoorthy Kuppusamy MBBS MD DM
Senior Consultant Neurologist
The Brain, Spine and Nerve Centre
Chennai, Tamil Nadu, India

Krishnaprasad TP MBBS MD DM
Consultant Neurologist
Krishna Neuro Centre
Karur, Tamil Nadu, India

Lenin Sankar Palanisamy MD
Resident
Institute of Neurology
Madras Medical College
Chennai, Tamil Nadu, India

Madhavi Karri MD MBBS
Neurology Resident
Department of Neurology
PSG Institute of Medical Sciences and Research
Coimbatore, Tamil Nadu, India

Manjeera Sri Padma K MBBS MD DM
Senior Resident
Department of Neurology
Nizams Institue of Medical Sciences (NIMS)
Hyderabad, Telangana, India

Mariappan V MBBS MD
Resident
Institute of Neurology
Madras Medical College
Chennai, Tamil Nadu, India

Meena A Kanikannan MD DM
Professor
Department of Neurology
Nizam's Institute of Medical Sciences
Hyderabad, Telangana, India

Contributors

Mini Sreedharan MD DM
Additional Professor
Department of Paediatric Neurology
Government Medical College
Thiruvananthapuram, Kerala, India

Muralidharan Nair MD DM
Professor (Senior Grade)
Department of Neurology
Sree Chitra Tirunal Institute for Medical
Sciences and Technology
Thiruvananthapuram, Kerala, India

Namrata Jayaharan MBBS MD
Resident, Institute of Neurology
Madras Medical College
Chennai, Tamil Nadu, India

Parvathy Rajan MSc
Scientific Assistant
Neuroimmunology Laboratory
Department of Neurology
Amrita Institute of Medical Sciences
Ponekkara, Kochi, Kerala, India

Sarala Govindarajan MBBS MD DM
Professor of Neurology
Institute of Neurology
Madras Medical College
Chennai, Tamil Nadu, India

Saranya Masilamani MBBS MD
Resident
Institute of Neurology
Madras Medical College
Chennai, Tamil Nadu, India

Sindhuja Lakshminarasimhan MBBS MD DNB DM
Consultant Neurologist
Institute of Neurology
Madras Medical College
Chennai, Tamil Nadu, India

Sireesha Yareeda MD DM
Assistant Professor
Department of Neurology
Nizam's Institute of Medical Sciences
Hyderabad, Telangana, India

Soumya Sundaram MD DM
Assistant Professor
Department of Neurology
Sree Chitra Tirunal Institute for Medical
Sciences and Technology
Thiruvananthapuram, Kerala, India

Sreenivas Umaiorubahan Meenakshisundaram MD
Resident
Institute of Neurology
Madras Medical College
Chennai, Tamil Nadu, India

Srinivasan Avathvadi Venkatesan MD DM FAAN FIAN FRCP (London) PhD DSc
Emeritus Professor
The Tamil Nadu Dr. M.G.R. Medical University
Adjunct Professor, Indian Institute of Technology (IIT - Chennai)
Chennai, Tamil Nadu, India

Sruthi S Nair MD DM
Assistant Professor
Department of Neurology
Sree Chitra Tirunal Institute for Medical
Sciences and Technology
Thiruvananthapuram, Kerala, India

Sudheeran Kannoth MD DM
Clinical Assistant Professor
Neuroimmunology Laboratory
Department of Neurology
Amrita Institute of Medical Sciences
Ponekkara, Kochi, Kerala, India

Sujin Koshy MBBS MD DM
Junior Consultant Neurologist
Believers Church Medical College Hospital
Thiruvalla, Kerala, India

Syam Krishnan Nair MBBS MD DM
Additional Professor
Department of Neurology
Sree Chitra Tirunal Institute for Medical
Sciences and Technology
Thiruvananthapuram, Kerala, India

Tushar VP MBBS MD
Institute of Neurology
Madras Medical College
Chennai, Tamil Nadu, India

Venkateswaran Kuttuva Jeyaram
MBBS MD
Resident, Institute of Neurology
Madras Medical College
Chennai, Tamil Nadu, India

Yashodara Priyadarshini MBBS
Medical Officer
IJ Multispecialty and Neuro Hospital
Chennai, Tamil Nadu, India

Foreword

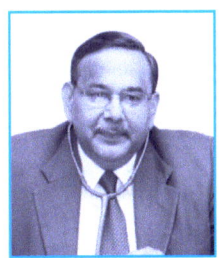

Rohini Handa MD DNB FAMS FICP FRCP (Glasgow)
Dean, Indian College of Physicians
Honorary Consultant Rheumatology, Armed Forces Medical Services
Quondam
Professor of Medicine, All India Institute of Medical Sciences, New Delhi
President APLAR (Asia Pacific League of Associations for Rheumatology)
President Indian Rheumatology Association

Senior Consultant Rheumatologist
Indraprastha Apollo Hospitals
New Delhi, India

Neurologic disorders are commonly encountered by all physicians and constitute an important chunk of internal medicine practice. Autoimmunity is increasingly being identified as the culprit pathobiologic process in a variety of neurologic diseases, particularly those affecting the peripheral nervous system. Immune dysregulation also underlies multiple sclerosis, myasthenia gravis, some myopathies and paraneoplastic syndromes. The list continues to expand. This monograph reviews recent developments in our understanding of the pathophysiology, clinical presentations and diagnoses of selected immune-mediated neurological disorders. Immunotherapy is also discussed.

Prof K Mugundhan, Drs R Lakshmi Narasimhan and Rajesh Shankar Iyer have assembled a galaxy of distinguished authors to cover all facets of this esoteric, and at times mysterious, field. The subject is contemporary and the concepts rapidly changing and evolving. This authoritative work is likely to appeal to the discerning reader interested in this fascinating field!

Foreword

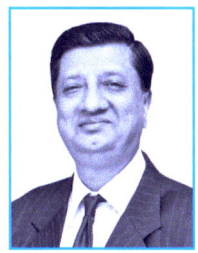

Sudhir V Shah MD DM (Neurology)
Professor and Head of Department
NHL MMC and SVPIMSR
Ahmedabad, Gujarat, India
and Director of Neurosciences
Sterling Hospital
Ahmedabad, Gujarat, India

It is a matter of immense pleasure that I am writing the foreword to this book—"Immune-mediated Neurological Disorders" edited by Dr Lakshmi Narasimhan Ranganathan, Dr Mugundhan Krishnan, and Dr Rajesh Shankar Iyer. The multilayered immune architecture in our body provides exemplary defense against the invisible microbes. However, disease ensues when the immune errands err and go haywire as exemplified by the process of autoimmunity. Paul Ehrlich in 1901 had theorized the concept and process of autoimmunity, and had coined the term "horror autotoxicus". The field has evolved ever since and has witnessed advancements in pathogenesis, scientists toiling with newer autoantibodies, and discovery of targeted therapies. Unraveling the mysteries of autoimmunity has unearthed answers to the enigmas that had long been left unanswered. The evolution of advanced laboratory techniques has resulted in the revelation of newer autoantibodies. However, it is of utmost importance to establish the pathogenic nature of such antibodies in the given constellation of symptoms of the presenting patient.

In the current scenario of rapidly expanding information in the field of autoimmunity in neurology, this book, *Immune-mediated Neurological Disorders*, is very valuable in organizing the vast information and is the need. There are very few books on autoimmunity in neurology, which are clear, comprehensive, and complete. Meeting these demands, the book has been beautifully scripted with chapters focusing on the spectrum of neurological presentations associated with various antibodies, the approach to autoimmune syndrome in a patient with specific neurological presentation, and the final chapter on immunotherapy crowns the masterpiece. The chapters are excellently written with suitable information crisply condensed in Tables, Flowcharts, and Images. The salient points are suitably summarized at the end of the chapter and help the resident in rapid revision and a busy practitioner with maximum information at a minimum glance.

This book is an important addition to the medical armamentarium of the residents, practicing neurologists, and academicians in knowing the autoimmune spectrum of disorders in neurology. Further, tailoring the book to the needs of our part of the world adds value to the book. I strongly recommend the book to all residents, physicians, neurologists, and those with interest in autoimmunity and congratulate the editors and authors on completing the monumental work.

Preface

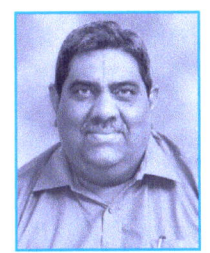

Lakshmi Narasimhan Ranganathan

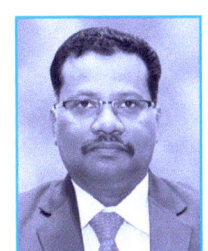

Mugundhan Krishnan

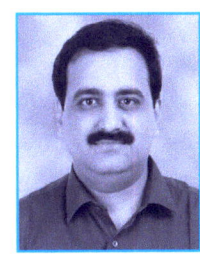

Rajesh Shankar Iyer

Neurology has been once plagued by therapeutic nihilism. However over the last three decades, various breath taking developments happened in the field of neurology which have not only put an end to nihilism, but has made it the most interesting and attractive specialty all over the world. Rapid development of diagnostic and therapeutic strategies has made life easy for people with stroke and epilepsy. Similarly autoimmune neurology is another specialty which has developed by leaps and bounds. It is called the 21st century subspecialty of neurology. Autoimmune neurology is unique in that it has a bearing on all subspecialties of neurology including cognitive neurology, epilepsy, movement disorders, spinal cord disorders, and muscle and peripheral nerve disorders and so on.

In this monograph, we take you through the various autoimmune disorders of the nervous system. After a brief introduction to the subject in the first chapter, we try to elaborate the various neural antibodies which helped us understand the disease in the second and then move on to their laboratory diagnosis in the third. In the subsequent five chapters, we discuss the autoimmune disorders affecting the upper storey including the dementias, demyelinating diseases, epilepsies, movement disorders and the cerebellar ataxias. A brief outline about the autoimmune myelopathies in the ninth chapter is followed by a sojourn into the lower storey and we see how the disorder affects the peripheral nerves, neuromuscular junction and the muscle in the subsequent three chapters. Finally we look into the various treatment options available and the current guidelines.

We have conceived the topics with the idea of providing the treating physician a comprehensive overview of this fast developing and fascinating subspecialty of neurology. It is imperative that we develop a high index of suspicion and look for the antibodies in the appropriate clinical setting and initiate immunotherapy at the earliest so that the dreaded sequelae are avoided. We hope that our efforts are a positive step in this direction.

Wishing you all a Happy and Enjoyable Reading!

Lakshmi Narasimhan Ranganathan
Mugundhan Krishnan
Rajesh Shankar Iyer

Contents

1. **Introduction** — 1
   Madhavi Karri, Rajesh Shankar Iyer

2. **Anti-neural Antibodies and the Disease Associations** — 5
   *Balasubramanian Samivel, Venkateswaran Kuttuva Jeyaram,
   Kaushik MG, Krishnamoorthy Kuppusamy, Lakshmi Narasimhan Ranganathan*

3. **Laboratory Evaluation of Neuronal Antibodies** — 22
   Annamma Mathai, Davidson Devasia, Parvathy Rajan, Sudheeran Kannoth

4. **Autoimmune Dementia** — 27
   *Lakshmi Narasimhan Ranganathan, Arun Shivaraman Mulanur Murugesan,
   Lenin Sankar Palanisamy, Sreenivas Umaiorubahan Meenakshisundaram,
   Kannan Vangiliappan, Guhan Ramamurthy, Srinivasan Avathvadi Venkatesan*

5. **Autoimmune Demyelinating Disorders** — 39
   *Mugundhan Krishnan, Lakshmi Narasimhan Ranganathan,
   Chandramouleeswaran V, Mariappan V, Balasubramanian Samivel,
   Ganesh Veeraraghavan*

6. **Autoimmune Epilepsies** — 53
   Afshan Jabeen Shaik, Manjeera Sri Padma K

7. **Autoimmune Movement Disorders** — 67
   Syam Krishnan Nair

8. **Autoimmune Cerebellar Ataxias** — 76
   Sujin Koshy, Rajesh Shankar Iyer

9. **Autoimmune Myelopathies** — 84
   Mini Sreedharan, Kalpana D

10. **Immune-mediated Neuropathies** — 93
    Meena A Kanikannan, Sireesha Yareeda

11. **Autoimmune Disorders of the Neuromuscular Junction** — 110
    *Sarala Govindarajan, Harish Jayakumar, Yashodara Priyadarshini,
    Lakshmi Narasimhan Ranganathan, Sindhuja Lakshminarasimhan, Tushar VP*

12. **Autoimmune Myopathy** — 121
    *Mugundhan Krishnan, Lakshmi Narasimhan Ranganathan,
    Jawahar Marimuthu, Krishnaprasad TP, Saranya Masilamani, Namrata Jayaharan*

13. **Immunotherapy** — 129
    Sruthi S Nair, Soumya Sundaram, Muralidharan Nair

PLATE 1

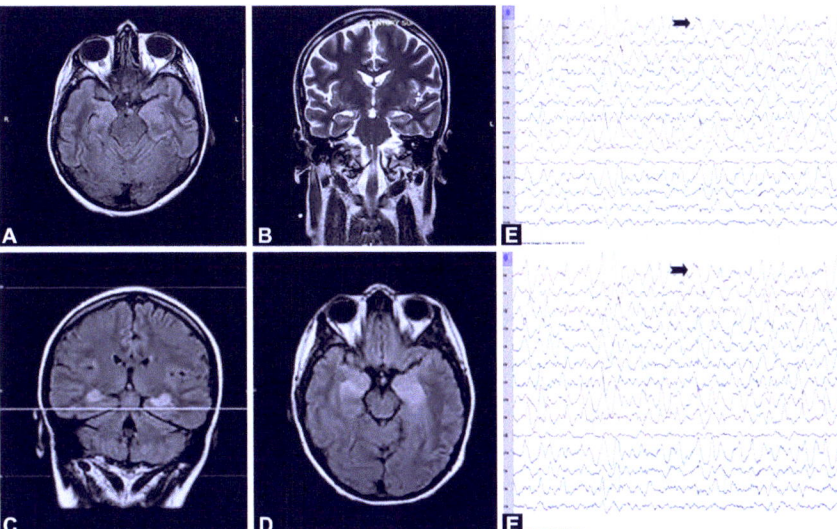

Note: She was also having a small ovarian teratoma but could not be operated in view of poor general condition.

FIG. 1: A 23-year-old lady presented with fever followed by seizures and abnormal behavior. Her initial MRI Brain **A** and **B,** was normal. She was diagnosed as viral meningoencephalitis and treated empirically with acyclovir and antipsychotics. She developed orofacial dyskinesias which were thought to be drug induced and antipsychotics were stopped. Slowly she became mute, developed dysautonomia and hypoventilation for which she was intubated and brought to our hospital. Repeat MRI Brain **C** and **D,** showed bilateral mesial temporal hyperintensities and EEG **E,** demonstrated extreme delta brushes (solid arrow). A diagnosis of NMDA receptor encephalitis was made. Serum and CSF both were showing NMDA receptor antibodies. Patient was treated with steroids and IVIG without any clinical response. Second line immunotherapy with rituximab was given. Patient succumbed to the illness secondary to severe respiratory tract infection. *(Chapter 6)*

PLATE 2

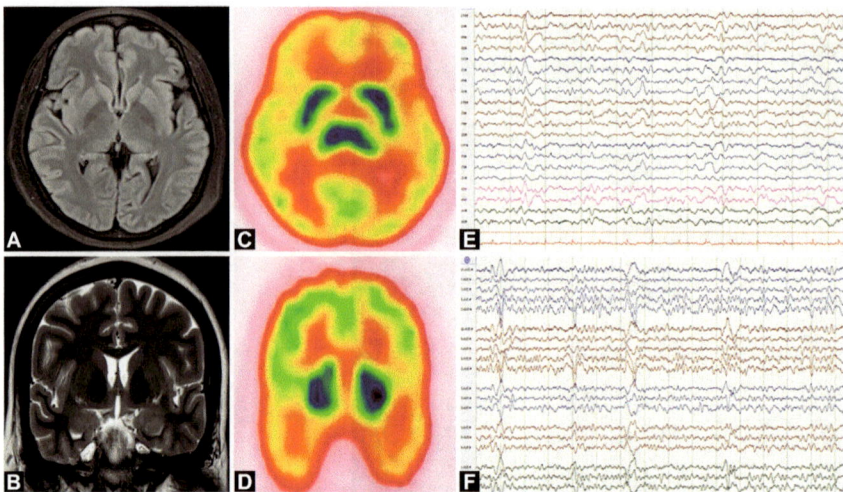

FIG. 2: A 38-year-old lady presented with low grade fever for 2 weeks followed by psychiatric disturbances in the form of delusions and hallucinations, 3 episodes of GTCS and infrequent myoclonus. Neurological examination revealed impaired memory and executive dysfunction. MRI Brain **A** and **B**, was normal. CT PET scan **C** and **D**, showed Bilateral basal ganglionic hypermetabolism. EEG **E** and **F**, revealed diffuse theta to delta range slowing. CSF analysis was normal. Serum and CSF analysis for antibodies (onconeural and ANSA) were negative. She was emperically treated with steroids with which she had a dramatic improvement. A diagnosis of Autoimmune encephalitis was made in the absence of antibodies. *(Chapter 6)*

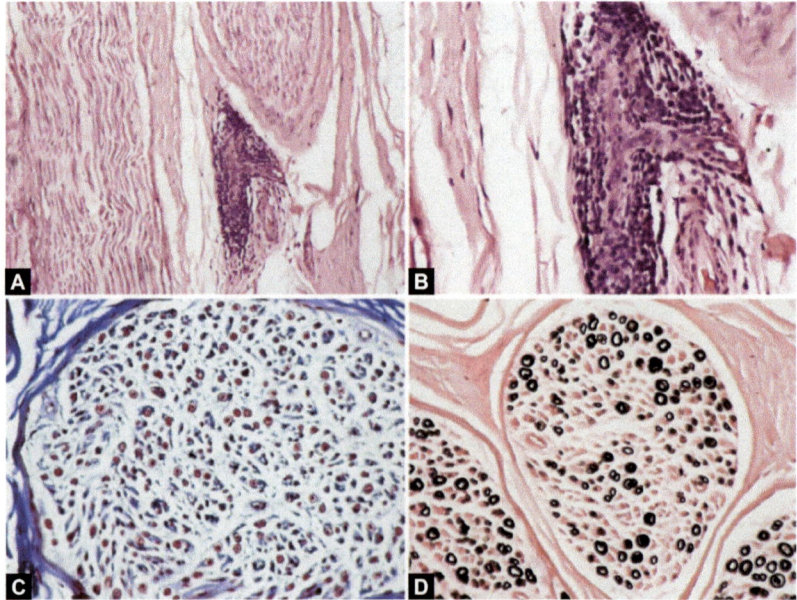

FIG. 2: A and B, Presence of perivascular lymphocytic infiltrate with vascular wall destruction; C, Increase in endoneurial collagen (MTX40 D, Sectorial multifocal nonuniform fiber loss (KpalX40). *(Chapter 10)*

CHAPTER 1

Introduction

Madhavi Karri, Rajesh Shankar Iyer

INTRODUCTION

Autoimmune neurology is one of the rapidly evolving fields in the modern neurology with focal autoimmune target (involvement) of central and peripheral nervous system. They are often subacute onset of illness with multifocal symptoms. It usually affects 5–10% of general population. Early identification of the disease is usually challenging. There has been tremendous advancement in evolution of autoimmune neurology in past one decade with newer techniques for identification of neural specific antibody profiles.

HISTORIC BACKGROUND

Antibody mediated neurological illness were first identified in mid-1970s but has gained momentum in the last decade in view of rapid modernization. The presence of neural specific antibody is often associated with neurologic syndrome. Newer diagnostic modalities have been identified not only for evaluation and diagnosis of autoimmune syndromes but also helped in treatment approach and therapeutic decision making.

EPIDEMIOLOGY AND PATHOPHYSIOLOGY

Neuroimmunology can target any structure of nervous system—both central and peripheral. There is a complex interplay between the immune system, genetic process and environmental factors. If there is underlying positive family history or malignancy it can heighten the suspicion of neuroimmunological pathology. B-cells act as precursors of antibody producing cells and also play a role in regulation of T-cell activation process. Several pathological mechanisms are considered to play a role in evolution of the varied diseases. The associated antibodies are targeted against either intracellular antigens which include anti-Hu, Ma2, CV2/collapsin response mediator protein 5 which are classical for paraneoplastic diseases, or cell membrane antigens like voltage gated potassium channels, N-methyl-D-aspartate receptor, α-amino-3-hydroxy-5-methyl-4-isoxazolepropionic acid receptor antibody which bind competitively to the target receptor and blocks the function of receptor, or they internalize and reduce the number of surface receptors thereby reducing the receptor activation. This binding may at times lead to cellular or complement mediated cytotoxicity as in neuromyelitis optica (NMO). Another variant of immune mechanism which targets cytoplasmic enzyme is glutamate decarboxylase 65 (GAD65) antibody.

Disease spectrum concerned with intracellular antigens are often associated with malignancies which trigger the autoimmune response (also called as paraneoplastic) and have a poor response to treatment and poor prognosis. Whereas others associated with cell mediated antibodies are usually considered as nonparaneoplastic and have better response to treatment.

CLINICAL SPECTRUM

Autoimmune neurologic disorder is characterized by detection of objective neurological deficit of subacute onset, presence of neural specific antibody, and its improvement with immunotherapy. The spectrum of autoimmune neurology includes autoimmune epilepsies, autoimmune dementias and demyelinating diseases, autoimmune movement disorders, autoimmune cerebellar ataxias, autoimmune neuromuscular junction disorders, autoimmune myelopathies, and peripheral neuropathies and myopathies.

WORKUP

Traditionally, it was considered as one among the rare disorders that evaluation for the same was unwarranted few decades ago. In the last decade, there has been tremendous evolvement of newer diagnostic modalities for the detection of novel antibodies and associated clinical phenotypes (Table 1). Usually they are diagnosed on the basis of typical clinical syndrome and supportive findings which include presence of neural antibody, magnetic resonance imaging or cerebrospinal fluid (CSF) analysis. Isolated antibody test results should never be taken into consideration.

Unless high degree of suspicion for specific disease like NMO where single antibody testing can be given, usually global antibodies screening has been advised. Identification of neural antibodies either in serum or CSF or both are very crucial. Immunohistochemistry and indirect tissue immunofluorescence are very important screening tools in identification of neural antibodies. Serum or CSF of the individuals who are to be tested is incubated. Immunohistochemistry helps in localization of specific antigens in tissue by use of markers and their binding patterns. Cell-based assays usually have higher specificity. Cell membrane antibodies are more difficult to test but have higher sensitivity and specificity with CSF.

Enzyme-linked immunosorbent assay test uses incubated serum or CSF with purified target attached to the walls of the plate. They are rapid and easily available tests. Only disadvantage is higher chance of false positives. Western blot is useful for identification of antibodies attached to cytosolic or nuclear antigens. Radioimmunoprecipitation assays are used for assessing ion channel antibodies. It is used for quantification analysis of the pathogenic antigen which is precipitated by antihuman immunoglobulin G.

Cerebrospinal fluid testing has an additional role in suspected autoimmune neurologic pathology. Ideally paired serum and CSF samples are taken for testing. Usually seen in NMO where NMDA receptor antibody is positive in CSF can have serum negativity in about of 8% of individuals. In serum positive individuals, there is definite CSF positivity for the antibody.

Evaluation for systemic malignancy in presence of paraneoplastic antibodies. Presence of paraneoplastic antibodies has strong positive predictive value for tumor existence. Identification of underlying tumor is useful for early treatment of relevant tumor and early tumor therapy with immune therapy.

Introduction

TABLE 1: Clinical clues in recognizing particular types and associated antibodies

Clinical features	Associated antibodies
Ptosis (mostly asymmetrical), diurnal variations, diplopia	Anti-AchR antibody, anti-MuSK antibody, anti-SM antibody, anti-LRP4 antibody
Acute ascending paralysis	Anti-GM1 antibody, anti-GQ1b antibody, anti-GD1a antibody
Myelopathies with or without optic neuritis	Aquaporin-4 antibodies, CRMP-5-IgG
Morvan's syndrome (neuromyotonia, muscle fasciculations, myokymia), Isaac's syndrome (cramps, fasciculations)	CASPR
Stiff person syndrome	GAD65, amphiphysin
Progressive encephalomyelitis with rigidity and myoclonus; hereditary hyperekplexia with exaggerated startle	Glycine receptor
Status epilepticus	NMDAR, GABA-A-R, GABA-B-R
Fasciobrachial dystonic seizures	LG1
Psychosis	NMDAR, GABA-B-R, AMPAR
Dystonia, chorea	Sydenham chorea, NMDAR
Cranial neuropathies	Miller-Fischer, Biskerstaff encephalitis
Myoclonus, startle, with gastrointestinal involvement	DPPX
Cerebellitis	ANNA-1, PCA-1, GAD65, VGCC

AchR, acetylcholine receptor; MuSK, muscle-specific kinase; SM, Smith; LRP4, lipoprotein receptor-related protein 4; CRMP-5, collapsin response-mediator protein-5; IgG, immunoglobulin G; GABA, γ-aminobutyric acid; NMDAR, N-methyl-D-aspartate receptor; AMPAR, α-amino-3-hydroxy-5-methyl-4-isoxazolepropionic acid receptor; CASPR5, contactin associated protein like 5; GAD65, glutamic acid decarboxylase 65 kDa; DPPX, dipeptidyl-peptidase-like protein-6; ANNA, anti-neuronal nuclear antibodies; PCA, purkinje cell cytoplasmic antibody; VGCC, voltage gated calcium channel; LG1, leucine-rich glioma-inactivated 1.

Magnetic resonance imaging of brain will be standard for identification of hyperintensities in T2-weighted images. Computed tomography thorax, abdomen and pelvis, mammogram, and ultrasonogram of testis are to be considered. Positron emission tomography can enhance the yield by 20% when all the above are inconclusive and is unaffected with treatment.

Electroencephalography is useful for identification of subclinical seizures and for particular diagnoses. It is also helpful in predicting the disease outcome and associated prognosis. Presence of seizures always indicates active disease. Brain or nerve biopsy have no clear evidence of its benefit.

TREATMENT STRATEGIES

Immunotherapy has a pivotal role. No proper therapeutic response to immunotherapy or in absence of antibody are known to require long-term immunotherapy. It typically consists of intravenous pulse steroids (ideally intravenous methylprednisolone) or intravenous immunoglobulin. Plasma exchange can be considered in those who are refractory or in contradiction to the above treatment. Those requiring long-term treatment, steroids for 6 months or steroid sparing agents like azathioprine and mycophenolate mofetil can be considered. Rituximab (CD-20 monoclonal antibody) has a role in all the above treatment modalities are resistant or contraindicated. Favorable response supports the diagnosis, whereas lack of treatment response needs re-evaluation.

CONCLUSION

Autoimmune neurology marks an emerging era in neurology with diversity in clinical manifestations. A high degree of suspicion is needed considering the clinical heterogeneity and sub-acute evolution of symptoms. Along with routine detailed history and clinical evaluation, testing for specific auto-antibodies helps in timely and accurate diagnosis. They are not rare and are often treatable and reversible. In this brief introductory chapter, we provide an overview of neuro-immunology and its recent developments, which are useful for early identification, treatment and prevention of future disability.

TAKE HOME MESSAGES

- Autoimmune neurology involves spectrum of disorders involving both central and peripheral nervous system
- It is a T-cell mediated immune response where B-cells act as precursors and also have a role in regulation of T-cell activation process
- Depending on associated antibodies they can be categorized as either paraneoplastic or nonparaneoplastic diseases
- Newer diagnostic modalities like immunohistochemistry and immunofluorescence had gained momentum in the past decade for identification of several neural specific antigens and syndromes associated, which is important for therapeutic decisions and prognostication
- Treatment usually includes steroids or intravenous immunoglobulin or plasmapheresis as first-line agents.

SUGGESTED READINGS

1. Lancaster E. The diagnosis and treatment of autoimmune encephalitis. J Clin Neurol. 2016;12(1):1-13.
2. Oliver Tobin W, Pittock SJ. Autoimmune neurology of the central nervous system. Continuum (Minneap Minn). 2017;23(3, Neurology of Systemic Disease):627-53.
3. Rosenfeld MR, Dalmau JO. Paraneoplastic disorders of the CNS and autoimmune synaptic encephalitis. Continuum (Minneap Minn). 2012;18(2):366-83.
4. Shapira Y, Agmon-Levin N, Shoenfeld Y. Defining and analyzing geoepidemiology and human autoimmunity. J Autoimmun. 2010;34(3):J168-77.

CHAPTER 2

Anti-neural Antibodies and the Disease Associations

Balasubramanian Samivel, Venkateswaran Kuttuva Jeyaram, Kaushik MG, Krishnamoorthy Kuppusamy, Lakshmi Narasimhan Ranganathan

INTRODUCTION

Neural antibodies are defined as antibodies that are targeted against neural antigens and produce neuronal injury due to T-cell mediated or antibody-mediated mechanisms. Neural antibodies are found to be associated with both physiological and pathological conditions. Pathologically, it can occur in both malignant and nonmalignant conditions. Initially in 1960s, immune-mediated mechanism was found to contribute to the pathogenesis of disease. Later in 1980s, by advent of immunohistochemical staining, antibodies were identified and these were related to neuronal cell and which in turn was associated with tumor. Detection of these autoantibodies helps in diagnosis of the disease and its further management. These antibodies are detected even before the appearance of tumor. In this chapter, we briefly describe the classification and pathogenesis of neuronal antibodies and its disease association.

CLASSIFICATION

Classification of autoantibodies is based on:
- Autoimmunity in nervous system
- Physiological and pathological origin
- Antigenic target location
- Association with malignancies and nonmalignancies.

Autoimmunity in Nervous System

Autoimmunity is defined as development of an immune response against one's own cells and tissues due to either failure of recognition of own cells or upregulation of expression of body's own cell. Autoimmunity in nervous system is classified on the basis of glial and neuronal autoimmunity (Flowchart 1). The advent of glial autoimmunity in pathogenesis of disease resulted in new treatment strategies in nervous system. For example, discovery of aquaporin-4 (AQP4) antibodies in pathogenesis of neuromyelitis optica (NMO) spectrum disorders paved the way for differentiating it from multiple sclerosis in pathogenesis, diagnosis, management, and predicting the outcome. The neuronal autoimmunity results in neuronal loss and dysfunction which results in encephalitis, dementia, and seizures.

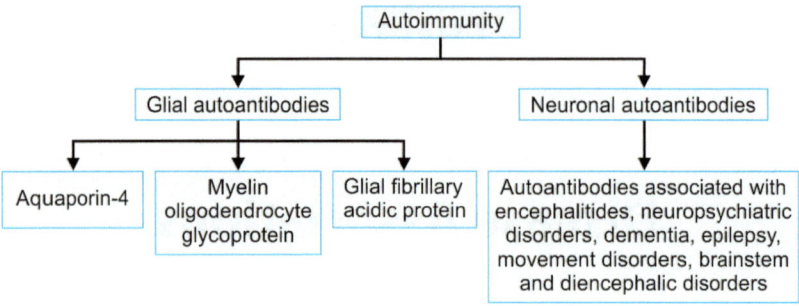

FLOWCHART 1: Autoimmunity in nervous system.

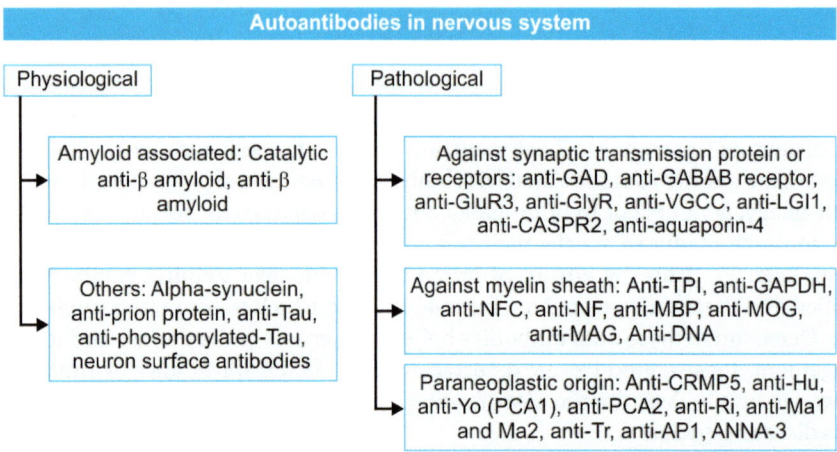

GAD, glutamic acid decarboxylase; GABA, gamma amino butyric acid; LGI1, leucine-rich glioma-inactivated 1; CASPR2, contactin-associated protein-like 2; TPI, triosephosphatisomerase; GAPDH, glyceraldehyde-3-phosphatedehydragenase; NFC, neurofascin; NF, neurofilament; MBP, myelin basic protein; MOG, myelin oligodendrocyte glycoprotein; MAG, myelin associated glycoprotein; DNA, deoxyribonucleic acid; CRMP5, collapsin response mediator protein 5; PCA, purkinje cell cytoplasmic antibody; AP1, Activator protein 1; ANNA-3, anti-neuronal nuclear antibodies-3.

FLOWCHART 2: Classification of autoantibodies based on physiological and pathological origin.

Physiological and Pathological Origin

The autoantibodies are classified on the basis of physiological and pathological origin (Flowchart 2). The physiological (naturally occurring) autoantibodies are involved in brain homeostasis and help in clearing the protein aggregates. The pathological autoantibodies are mostly of paraneoplastic origin and some are associated with nonparaneoplastic origin.

Antigenic Target Location

The autoantibodies are classified on the basis of targets at which they act and classified into synaptic and nonsynaptic (Flowchart 3). The synaptic autoantibodies act either intracellularly or extracellularly.

Non synaptic and synaptic autoantibodies

Nonsynaptic
- Anti-Hu, anti-CRMP5, anti-Ma1 and Ma2, anti-Yo, anti-Ri, anti-Tr, anti-zic4, anti-gephyrin, anti-GABA receptor associated protein

Synaptic autoantibodies
- Intracellular: Anti-GAD65, anti-amphiphysin
- Extracellular: Anti-NMDAR, anti-LGI1, anti-contactin associated protein like 2, anti-GABAB receptor, anti-AMPAR, anti-P/Q type VGCC, anti-metabotropic glutamate receptor 1 and 2

CRMP5, collapsin response mediator protein 5; GABA, gamma amino butyric acid; GAD65, glutamic acid decarboxylase 65kDa; NMDAR, N-methyl-d-aspartate receptor; LGI1, leucine-rich glioma-inactivated 1; AMPAR, α-amino-3-hydroxy-5-methyl-4-isoxazolepropionic acid receptor; VGCC, voltage gated calcium channels; zic4, zinc finger protein 4.

FLOWCHART 3: Classification of autoantibodies based on antigenic target location—synaptic and nonsynaptic target antigens.

Based on association with malignant and nonmalignant conditions

Cytosolic/nuclear antibodies
- Anti-ANNA 1(Hu), anti-ANNA 2(Ri), anti-ANNA 3, anti-Ma1/Ma2, anti-CV2/CRMP5, anti-PCA1,PCA2, anti-ARHGAP26, anti-Zic4, anyi-SOX1, anti-titin, anti-recoverin

Intracellular synaptic antibodies
- Anti-amphiphsin, anti-GAD65

Surface antibodies
- Anti-AQ4, anti-NMDAR, anti-AMPAR, anti-LGI1, anri-CASPR2, anti-GABAB receptor, anti-GABAA receptor, anti-DR2

ANNA, anti-neuronal nuclear antibodies; CRMP5, collapsin response mediator protein 5; PCA, purkinje cell cytoplasmic antibody; ARHGAP26, Rho GTPase activating protein 26; GAD65, glutamic acid decarboxylase 65kDa; NMDAR, N-methyl-d-aspartate receptor; AQ4, aquaporin 4; AMPAR, α-amino-3-hydroxy-5-methyl-4-isoxazolepropionic acid receptor; LGI1, leucine-rich glioma-inactivated 1; CASPR2, contactin-associated protein-like 2; GABA, gamma amino butyric acid.

FIG. 1: Classification of autoantibodies based on association with malignant and nonmalignant conditions.

Association with Malignancies and Nonmalignancies

Most of the autoantibodies described are of paraneoplastic origin and these antibodies act at different levels to produce various manifestations (Fig. 1). The antibodies acting on cell surface antigens may be paraneoplastic or most often nonparaneoplastic, whereas the antibodies against the nuclear or cytosolic antigens are mostly associated with malignant conditions. The neurological manifestations are described later in this chapter.

MECHANISM OF ANTIBODY-MEDIATED NEURONAL INJURY

Neural-specific antibody is often classically associated with a neurologic syndrome, the pathophysiology of which varies between diseases in situations like:
- Intracellular antigenic targets: The antibody is likely to be a marker of disease and is likely not to be pathogenic. In these cases, it is thought that the pathogenic agent is more likely the T-cell effector cell, which causes which cause irreversible injury due to T-cell mediated effects, and these are usually associated with malignancy and show poor response to treatment
- In contrast, antibody directed against cell surface antigens most often occurs in young individuals, may or may not be associated with cancer. They are directly pathogenic and produce distinct clinical syndromes which show good response to immunotherapy.

Pathogenesis of Neural Antibodies

Tumor-related Antibodies

Neural injury is mainly due to tumor-mediated immune response which is initiated by onconeural proteins. These proteins are expressed in plasma membrane, nucleus, nucleolus, and cytoplasm of neural cells. Antigens in these sites are presented to adaptive immunity and results in activation of immune system leading to multiple effector mechanism [Immunoglobulin G (IgG) mediated or T-cell mediated] (Flowchart 4).

The Effector Mechanism

- Effector mechanism is different in the case of intracellular and cell surface antigens
- The mechanism of neuronal injury is mediated through T-cell in intracellular antigens, whereas it is antibody mediated with respect to cell surface antigens (Fig. 2).

Effector Mechanism for Cell Surface and Membrane Antigens

- Antibody targets the antigens on plasma cell membrane and acts as effectors of injury

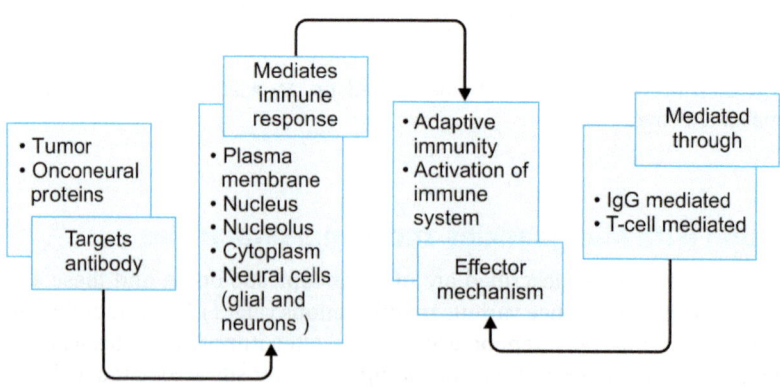

FLOWCHART 4: Pathogenesis of neural antibodies.

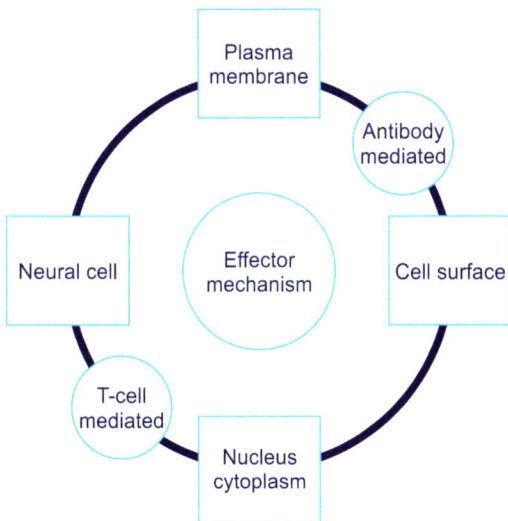

FIG. 2: Effector mechanism.

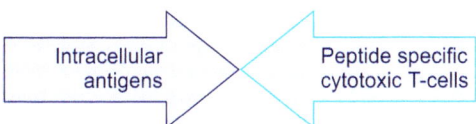

FIG. 3: Effector mechanism of intracellular antigens.

- Antibody targeting on neural cell membrane acts on various channels [voltage-gated potassium channel (VGKC), N-methyl-d-aspartate (NMDA), alpha-amino-3-hydroxy-5-methyl-4-isoxazole-propionic acid (AMPA), gamma amino butyric acid (GABA)-B, AQP4] which leads to cell dysfunction
- Alteration or modulation of cell surface antigen by the neural antibodies activates various channels and produces damage in different ways like:
  - Receptor agonist or antagonist effects
  - Activation of complement cascade
  - Activation of Fc receptor: Leading to antibody-dependent cell-mediated cytotoxicity
  - Antigen internalization (Antigenic modulation): Alters the antigen density on the cell surface.

Effector Mechanism for Intracellular Antigens

Intracellular antigenic proteins (neural or cytoplasmic) undergo proteasomal degradation into peptides which are exposed to immune system through upregulation of major histocompatibility complex class I. These are then recognized by cytotoxic T-cells in a proinflammatory cytokine environment leading to T-cell activation and neural injury. Effector mechanism of injury is mainly mediated through peptide-specific cytotoxic T-cells (Fig. 3).

ANTINEURONAL ANTIBODIES AND ITS DISEASE ASSOCIATION

Classically, antineuronal antibodies are divided into two groups based on the target antigen.
- Nonsynaptic antibodies which include intracellular nuclear and cytoplasmic antibodies
- Synaptic antibodies which again divide into intracellular synaptic antibodies and extracellular or surface antibodies.

Nuclear and Cytoplasmic Antibodies

Antibodies against nuclear and cytoplasmic target antigen are nonpathogenic. They directly do not produce lethal affect. Presence of antibodies in cerebrospinal fluid (CSF) or serum acts as a marker for cancer. Possible mechanism by which these antibodies produce disorders is T-cell mediated response. For example, presence of Hu antibodies in small cell lung cancer. Expression of Hu is triggered by T-cell mediated autoimmune response. Various nonsynaptic antibodies and its associated syndromes are described in Table 1.

Intracellular Synaptic Antibodies

Intracellular synaptic antibodies are glutamic acid decarboxylase 65(GAD65) and amphiphysin. Glutamic acid decarboxylase 65 is concentrated in presynaptic terminals. Amphiphysins are proteins belonging to Bin-Amphiphysin-Rvs167 superfamily, which are important for recycling of vesicles in synaptic terminal through endocytosis mediated by clathrin. The pathological effects of GAD65 are through both antibody-mediated and T-cell mediated mechanisms (Table 2).

Cell-surface and Synaptic Antigens

Recently, large number of synaptic or cell surface antibodies are identified. The pathological effect of these antibodies is similar to disruption in the function of target antigen. Various cell surface and synaptic antibodies and their association with various syndromes are shown in Table 3.

CLINICAL PHENOTYPE-BASED APPROACH TO AUTOIMMUNE ANTIBODIES

Anti-neural antibodies produce various syndromes based on the target of action. It may be predominately peripheral or central syndromes. Based on clinical phenotype of various syndromes, they are divided into paraneoplastic syndromes or classic syndromes and idiopathic or nonclassic syndromes. Paraneoplastic syndromes are almost associated with malignancy and idiopathic syndromes do not have any evidence for malignancy (Table 4).

CLINICAL PRESENTATIONS OF ANTINEURAL ANTIBODIES WITH CENTRAL NERVOUS SYSTEM INVOLVEMENT

These are divided into:
- Autoimmune encephalitis
- Autoimmune dementia and neuropsychiatric disorders

TABLE 1: Nonsynaptic antibodies and associated disorders

Antibody	Antigen and mechanism	Associated tumor	Clinical constellation
Anti-Hu	• Hu proteins (HuD, HuC and Hel-N1, N2) • Neuronal RNA handling • T-cell mediated	Small cell lung cancer	Sensory neuropathy, limbic encephalitis, cerebellitis and brainstem encephalitis
Anti-Yo	• Yo proteins (CDR1 in Purkinje cells)t • CDR2 in cell cycle regulation and transcriptional regulation • Possibly T-cell mediated	Breast and gynecological malignancy	Paraneoplastic cerebellar degeneration
Anti-Ri	• Ri proteins (Nova 1 and Nova 2) • Nova 1 RNA binding protein • Antibodies inhibit binding of Nova 1 to RNA	Breast cancer	Paraneoplastic cerebellar degeneration, opsoclonus-myoclonus syndrome, encephalitis, and myelitis
Anti-CRMP5	• CRMP5 • Neurogenesis and its regulation • T-cell mediated	Small cell lung cancer, thymoma	Polyneuropathy, limbic encephalitis, cerebellar degeneration and uveoretinal syndrome
Anti-Ma	• Ma proteins (Ma1 and Ma2) • Ma1- apoptosis regulation • T-cell mediated	• Ma1–skin, lung, renal and gastrointestinal cancer • Ma2–germ cell tumors	Limbic encephalitis, cerebellitis, brainstem encephalitis and neuropathy
Anti-Tr	Tr proteins in Purkinje cells	Hodgkin lymphoma	Paraneoplastic cerebellar degeneration
Anti-gephyrin	• Gephyrin • Involved in GABAergic transmission	Mediastinal carcinoma	Stiff person syndrome
Anti-ZIC4	• Zinc finger protein • Mostly nonpathogenic	Small cell lung cancer	Paraneoplastic cerebellar degeneration

CDR, complementarity determining region; RNA, ribonucleic acid; CRMP5, collapsin response mediator protein 5; GABA, gamma amino butyric acid; ZIC4, zinc finger protein 4.

- Autoimmune epilepsy
- Diencephalic and brainstem disorders
- Immune-mediated movement disorders
- Autoimmune myelopathies
- Aquaporin-4 autoimmunity
- Myelin oligodendrocyte glycoprotein (MOG) autoimmunity
- Glial fibrillary acidic protein (GFAP) autoimmunity
- Stiff person syndrome
- Progressive encephalomyelitis with rigidity and myoclonus
- Autoimmune cerebellopathies.

TABLE 2: Intracellular synaptic antibodies and its associated disorders

Antibody	Antigen and mechanism	Associated tumor	Clinical constellation
Anti-amphiphysin	• Amphiphysin-synaptic vesicles recycling • Pathogenic	Breast cancer	Stiff person syndrome
Anti-GAD65	• Glutamic acid decarboxylase • Important for GABA synthesis • T cell mediated and antibody mediated	Rarely neuroendocrine tumors	Cerebellitis, stiff person syndrome

GAD65, glutamic acid decarboxylase; GABA, gamma amino butyric acid.

TABLE 3: Cell surface antigens and its associated disorders

Antibody	Antigen and mechanism	Associated tumor	Clinical constellation
Anti-NMDAR	• NMDAR NR1 subunit is the primary target • Important for learning and memory • Antibodies cross link with NMDAR and internalization of receptors	Ovarian teratoma	Limbic encephalitis, psychiatric symptoms, catatonia, autonomic dysfunction
Anti-GABAB	• GABA B receptor • Primarily inhibits synaptic transmission	Small cell lung cancer	Limbic encephalitis, refractory seizures
Anti-AMPA	• AMPA receptor • Important for learning and memory	Breast and lung cancer, thymoma	Limbic encephalitis
Anti-LGI 1	• Leucine-rich glioma inactivated protein 1 • Secreted protein • Crucial role in regulation of presynaptic VGKC Kv1	None	Hyponatremia, limbic encephalitis, seizures or myoclonus
Anti-CASPR2	• Contactin associated protein 2 • Crucial role on organization of VGKC Kv1 channels	Thymoma	Limbic encephalitis, neuromyotonia
Anti-VGCC	• Voltage-gated calcium channels P/Q type • Important for presynaptic calcium influx • Pathogenic blocking of calcium influx	Small cell lung cancer	Lambert–Eaton myasthenia syndrome
Anti-metabotropic glutamate receptor	• Metabotropic glutamate receptor 1–important for cerebellar function	Hodgkin lymphoma	Cerebellitis
	• Metabotropic glutamate receptor 5–important for hippocampal function	Hodgkin lymphoma	Ophelia syndrome

NMDA, N-methyl-d-aspartate receptor; GABA, gamma amino butyric acid; AMPA, alpha-amino-3-hydroxy-5-methyl-4- isoxazole-propionic acid; LGI1, leucine-rich glioma-inactivated 1; CASPR2, contactin-associated protein-like 2; VGKC, voltage-gated potassium channel.

TABLE 4: Clinical phenotype-based approach

Site	Paraneoplastic syndrome	Idiopathic syndrome
Central nervous system	• Encephalomyelitis • Limbic encephalitis • Paraneoplastic cerebellar degeneration • Opsoclonus-myoclonus syndrome	• Brainstem encephalitis • Stiff person syndrome • Necrotizing myelopathy • Motor neuron disease
Dorsal root ganglia or peripheral nerves	• Subacute sensory neuronopathy • Gastrointestinal paresis or pseudo-obstruction	• Acute sensorimotor neuropathy (Guillain–Barre syndrome, plexitis) • Subacute and chronic sensorimotor neuropathies • Neuropathy of plasma cell dyscrasias and lymphoma • Pure autonomic neuropathy • Vasculitic neuropathies
Muscle	Dermatomyositis	• Acute necrotizing myopathy • Polymyositis
Neuromuscular junction	Lambert–Eaton myasthenia syndrome	• Myasthenia gravis • Acquired neuromyotonia
Eye and retina	• Cancer associated retinopathy • Melanoma associated retinopathy	Optic neuritis

Autoimmune Encephalitis

The presentation is usually a subacute onset of an encephalitic syndrome with altered sensorium, seizures, psychiatric disturbances, and movement disorders. Syndromes due to autoimmune encephalitis and due to autoimmune dementia and neuropsychiatric disorders are combined together because of frequent overlap (Table 5).

Autoimmune Epilepsy

Autoimmune epilepsy is suspected when the patient has any one of the following:
- Status epilepticus which is new onset
- Refractory status epilepticus
- Rapid cognitive decline
- Early age of onset (Table 6).

Autoimmune Myelopathy

Based on the course of the disorder, autoimmune myelopathies are divided into:
- Acute or subacute onset of motor, sensory, or autonomic spinal cord dysfunction
- Insidious onset and progressive course
- Motor neuron disease-like presentation (Table 7).

TABLE 5: Antibodies associated with autoimmune encephalitis

Syndrome	Antibodies	Associated cancer
Anti-NMDA receptor encephalitis	NMDA receptor	Ovarian teratoma
Limbic encephalitis	• AMPA receptor • GABAB receptor • LGI1 • CASPR2 • Hu (ANNA-1) • Ma2 • GAD	• Thymoma, small cell lung carcinoma • Small cell lung carcinoma • Thymoma • Thymoma • Small cell lung carcinoma • Testicular seminoma • Thymoma, small cell lung carcinoma
Encephalitis	• GABAA • mGLuR5 • DPPX	• Thymoma • Hodgkin's lymphoma • Lymphoma
Acute disseminated encephalomyelitis	MOG	–
Basal ganglia encephalitis	Dopamine 2 receptor	–
Bickerstaff's encephalitis	GQ1b	–
NMO spectrum disorder	Aquaporin 4	–

NMDA, N-methyl-d-aspartate; GABA, gamma amino butyric acid; AMPA, alpha-amino-3-hydroxy-5-methyl-4-isoxazole-propionic acid; MOG, myelin oligodendrocyte glycoprotein; LGI1, leucine-rich glioma-inactivated 1; CASPR2, contactin-associated protein-like 2; GAD, glutamic acid decarboxylase; ANNA, anti-neuronal nuclear antibodies; DPPX, dipeptidyl-peptidase-like protein-6; GQ1b, Ganglioside Q1b.

Autoimmune Neuropathy

Various phenotypic presentations of autoimmune neuropathy are:
- Sensory neuronopathy, most common
- Autonomic enteric neuropathy
- Demyelinating neuropathy
- Motor neuropathy very rare (Table 8).

Autoimmune Cerebellopathies

Cerebellar Purkinje cell proteins are target antigen for various antineural antibodies (Table 9).

Autoimmune Movement Disorder

They frequently occur in adults. Complete range of movement disorder phenotype is associated with autoimmune movement disorder. It may mimic a neurodegenerative disease. Antibodies associated with autoimmune movement disorder are shown in Table 10.

Autoimmune Neuromuscular Disorders

Autoimmune disorders of neuromuscular junction (NMJ) cause severe neurological impairment. The mechanism of NMJ failure could be destruction of normal structures

TABLE 6: Antibodies associated with autoimmune epilepsy

Various group	Syndromes	Antibodies
Paraneoplastic limbic encephalitis	Limbic encephalitis	Anti-Ma, mGluR5, CRMP5, amphiphysin, VGCC
Antibodies against VGKC channels	Limbic encephalitis	LGI1, CASPR2
NMDA encephalitis	Encephalitis	NMDAR
Rasmussen encephalitis	Encephalitis	GluR3
Other neuronal surface antigens	Limbic encephalitis	GABAA, GABAB, TPO, TG, SOX1
De novo febrile illness	• NORSE (new onset refractory status epilepticus) • FIRES (febrile infection related epilepsy syndrome) • AERRPS (acute encephalitis with refractory repetitive partial seizures)	None
Other autoimmune disorders	• ADEM • Nonconvulsive status • Epilepsia partialis continua	ADEM-anti MOG antibodies
Systemic autoimmune disorder	• SREAT (steroid responsive encephalopathy with autoimmune thyroiditis) • SLE	None

VGCC, voltage-gated calcium channel; SLE, systemic lupus erythematosus; NMDA, N-methyl-d-aspartate; GABA, gamma amino butyric acid; LGI1, leucine-rich glioma-inactivated 1; ADEM, acute disseminated encephalomyelitis; CASPR2, contactin-associated protein-like 2; VGKC, voltage-gated potassium channel; CRMP5, collapsin response mediator protein 5; TPO, thyroid peroxidase antibody; TG, Thyroglobulin; MOG, myelin oligodendrocyte glycoprotein.

which are responsible for function and transmission of signal or dysfunctional activity of same due to targeted mutation as seen in congenital myasthenic syndromes. Autoimmune NMJ disorders are classified as presynaptic and postsynaptic. Presynaptic antibodies are directed against voltage gated calcium channel in presynaptic terminals, thereby interfering with the presynaptic calcium influx required for acetylcholine release. In the paraneoplastic setting, 40% of cases are associated with small cell carcinoma of lung (SCLC). Around 3% patients with SCLC have Lambert–Eaton myasthenic syndrome (LEMS) that usually occurs in elderly. Other malignant conditions are Hodgkin's lymphoma, malignant thymoma and atypical carcinoid syndromes. Anti-SOX 1 is another presynaptic antibody implicated in paraneoplastic LEMS. In postsynaptic region, the antibodies are anti-MuSK, low density lipoprotein receptor-related protein family of transmembrane protein (LRP4), anti-rapsyn antibody, antibody targeted against non-AChR skeletal muscle proteins like anti-titin, anti-ryanodine, antibody against non-AChR ion channels like voltage-gated Kv1.4 is implicated.

Aquaporin-4 Autoimmunity

Aquaporin-4, a water channel protein, primarily located in astrocytes, is the target antigen in NMO spectrum disorder. Usually, NMO-IgG is not associated with any cancer. AQP4

TABLE 7: Common autoimmune myelopathies and its associated antibodies

Disease	Antibody	Cancer association	Course	Presentation
Multiple sclerosis	–	–	Relapsing	Subacute asymmetric
NMO	Aquaporin 4	–	Relapsing	Subacute symmetric
ADEM	MOG	–	Monophasic	Subacute multifocal with encephalitis
Paraneoplastic myelopathy	CRMP5 amphiphysin	Breast and lung carcinoma	Chronic progressive	Insidious
Autoimmune/ paraneoplastic motor neuron disease	Variable	Breast and lung carcinoma, lymphoma	Chronic progressive	• Mixed upper and lower motor neuron • ALS or PLS
Stiff person syndrome	Anti-GAD65 amphiphysin	Small cell lung cancer, thymoma	Chronic progressive	–
Progressive encephalomyelitis with rigidity and myoclonus	Anti-glycine receptor antibody	–	Subacute progressive	–

GAD, glutamic acid decarboxylase; NMO, neuromyelitis optica; MOG, myelin oligodendrocyte glycoprotein; ALS, amyotrophic lateral sclerosis; PLS, primary lateral sclerosis; ADEM, acute disseminated encephalomyelitis; CRMP5, collapsin response mediator protein 5.

is present in two major isoforms produced by alternative splicing: a relatively long (M1) isoform with translation initiation at Met-1, and a shorter (M23) isoform with translation initiation at Met-23. Aquaporin-4 monomers assemble as tetramers. The tetramers uniquely further aggregate in cell plasma membranes to form supramolecular assembles called orthogonal arrays of particles (OAPs) which were originally visualized in membranes by freeze-fracture electron microscopy. Aquaporin-4 is most strongly expressed in the central nervous system (CNS), but is also present in epithelial cells in the kidney (collecting duct), the stomach (parietal cells), airways, glands, and skeletal muscle. Aquaporin-4 is expressed in astrocytes in the brain, spinal cord, and optic nerve, and is particularly concentrated at pial and ependymal surfaces in contact with the CSF. At the cell level, AQP4 expression is polarized to foot processes of astrocytes in contact with blood vessels. Aquaporin-4 is also expressed in so-called supportive cells, similar to astrocytes in sensory organs such as Muller cells in the retina. Pathological changes associated with NMO mostly occur in the spinal cord and optic nerve, and to a lesser extent in the brain, with a notable absence of abnormalities in peripheral AQP4-expressing tissues.

Myelin Oligodendrocyte Glycoprotein Autoimmunity

Target protein in MOG autoimmunity is MOG belonging to immunoglobulin superfamily. It is expressed exclusively on the outer surface of myelin sheath and plasma membrane of the oligodendrocytes. Myelin oligodendrocyte glycoprotein is the most important surface

TABLE 8: Various antibodies associated with autoimmune neuropathy

Antibodies	Neuropathy	Malignancy
Nuclear or cytoplasmic		
Anti-Hu	• Sensory neuronopathy • Autonomic neuropathy • Motor neuropathy • Axonal sensorimotor neuropathy	• Small cell lung cancer • Neuroblastoma
Anti-CV2 (CRMP5)	• Peripheral neuropathy • Sensory neuronopathy • Optic neuropathy • Axonal sensorimotor neuropathy	Small cell lung cancer
Anti-Yo 1	Cerebellar ataxia, rarely motor neuropathy	• Ovarian cancer • Breast cancer
Anti-Ri	Sensorimotor neuropathy	• Breast cancer • Lung cancer
Amphiphysin	• Stiff person syndrome • Peripheral neuropathy	• Small cell lung cancer • Thymoma
Ion channel		
AChR antibodies—ganglionic nicotinic	Autonomic ganglionopathy	• Small cell lung cancer • Thymoma
Anti-VGKC	Autonomic neuropathy	• Small cell lung cancer • Thymoma
Anti-VGCC	Peripheral neuropathy	• Breast cancer • Lung cancer
Myelin associated glycoprotein (MAG) IgM	Sensorimotor neuropathy associated with paraproteinemia	• POEMS syndrome, Waldenstrom macroglobulinemia • Multiple myeloma
	Vasculitic neuropathy	Lymphoma
Anti-GM1 (IgM)	Multifocal motor neuropathy	–
Anti-GQ1b (IgG)	Miller Fisher syndrome	–
Anti-GM1, GD1a	Guillian-Barre syndrome	–
Anti-GD1b	• Chronic ataxic neuropathy with ophthalmoplegia • IgM paraprotein	–

POEMS, polyneuropathy, organomegaly, endocrinopathy, monoclonal protein, skin changes; VGCC, voltage-gated calcium channel; VGKC, voltage-gated potassium channel; CRMP5, collapsin response mediator protein 5.

marker of myelin for oligodendrocyte maturation. It forms only a minor component of myelin approximately 0.05%. Functions of MOG are regulation of microtubule stability, cell adhesion molecule and mediator between myelin and immune system. After various cell-based immune assays, high titer of MOG is associated with multiple sclerosis, acute disseminated encephalomyelitis, seronegative NMO or clinically isolated syndrome like optic neuritis or transverse myelitis. Myelin oligodendrocyte glycoprotein antibody titers are highly significant for pediatric age group as compared to adults.

TABLE 9: Following are the various antibodies and its associated syndromes

Antibody	Syndrome	Malignancy
Anti-Yo (PCA1)	Paraneoplastic cerebellar degeneration	Ovary and breast cancer
Anti-Hu	• PCD • Encephalomyelitis • Sensory neuronopathy	SCLC
Anti CV2	Limbic encephalitis, chorea, PCD	SCLC, thymoma
Anti-Ri	Opsoclonus-myoclonus syndrome Ataxia	Breast and ovarian cancer, SCLC
Tr	PCD	Hodgkin disease
ZIC4	PCD	SCLC
mGluR1	PCD	• Hodgkin lymphoma • Prostate adenocarcinoma
DNER	PCD	Hodgkin lymphoma
mGluR5	Ophelia syndrome	Hodgkin lymphoma

PCA, purkinje cell cytoplasmic antibody; PCD, paraneoplastic cerebellar degeneration; DNER, delta epidermal growth factor associated receptor.

TABLE 10: Antibodies associated with autoimmune movement disorder

Antibody	Syndrome
Anti-CRMP5	Chorea
Anti-Ma2	Rigidity and hypokinesia
Anti-LGI1	Chorea, myoclonus, tics
Anti-Yo	Tremor and cerebellar ataxia
Anti-Hu	Ataxia and pseudoathetosis
Anti-NMDAR	Dyskinesia, chorea, ballismus
CASPR2	Neuromyotonia
• GAD65 • Amphiphysin	Stiff person syndrome
Anti-Ri	Opsoclonus-myoclonus
• Antistreptolysin O, • Anti-desoxyribonuclease B • Anti-nicotinamide adenine dinucleotidase	Sydenham's chorea

CRMP, collapsin response mediator protein; NMDAR, N-methyl-d-aspartate receptor; GAD65, glutamic acid decarboxylase; CASPR2, contactin-associated protein-like 2; LGI1, leucine-rich glioma-inactivated 1.

Glial Fibrillary Acidic Protein Autoimmunity

Astrocytes are major type of glial cells in CNS. Astrocytes play an important role in homeostatic function of CNS. Astrocytes express a reactive phenotype in ischemia, CNS trauma and neurodegenerative disease. Glial fibrillary acidic proteins are the main intermediate filament proteins in astrocytes. They are upregulated in reactive phenotype of astrocytes. Recently, isoforms of GFAP are found to be a biomarker for steroid-responsive autoimmune meningoencephalomyelitis. Some neoplasms associated are gastroesophageal adenocarcinoma and prostrate carcinoma. Rarely, they are associated with myeloma, melanoma, and carcinoid tumor.

EVALUATION OF ANTIBODIES AND VARIOUS METHODS TO DETECT ANTIBODIES

Paired serum and CSF should be ideally tested in patients with suspected autoimmune disorder. Various methods to detect antibodies are indirect immunohistochemistry, western blot, radioimmunoprecipitation assay, cell-based assay and enzyme-linked immunosorbent assay. Nonsynaptic nuclear or cytoplasmic antibodies are best detected by western blot assay. Ion channel targeted antibodies are predominately detected by radioimmunoprecipitation assay. Cell-based assays are good to detect antibodies targeted against surface antigens. Through the immunohistochemistry method, most of the antibodies can be detected. Limitations for immunohistochemistry are presence of multiple antibodies and nonspecific binding of antibodies. Low titer antibodies are confirmed using western blot assay.

EVALUATION OF MALIGNANCY

Patients with positive family history of malignancy, risk factors like smoking or classical paraneoplastic syndromes should be evaluated extensively for malignancy. Following investigations help to identify associated malignancy; computed tomography scan of chest, abdomen, and pelvis; testicular ultrasound; mammography; and prostate-specific antigen. Diagnostic yield can be increased by positron emission tomography (PET) imaging when most of the diagnostic tests are negative. Drawback of PET imaging is low sensitivity in detecting gonadal tumors, neuroblastoma or thymoma. In such case, magnetic resonance imaging shows good sensitivity.

TREATMENT

Various treatment options available are intravenous (IV) methylprednisolone, IV immunoglobulin (IVIg) or plasma exchange. Intravenous methylprednisolone is considered as first line of treatment. In case patients who cannot tolerate IV steroids, IVIg can be used. In patient's refractory to treatment or contraindication with IV steroids and IVIg, plasma exchange can be tried. The duration and intensity of treatment depends on the severity of the clinical syndrome. Rapid escalation of treatment can be considered in clinically unstable patients who require intensive care support.

CONCLUSION

Neural antibodies have recently emerged as an important cause for central and peripheral nervous system dysfunction. These various neural antibodies are targeted against intracellular, nuclear, cytoplasmic antigens or against the cell surface antigens producing distinct clinical syndromes and disease association. Recognition of these antibodies and the clinical syndromes early in the course of the disease contribute to early intervention which thereby reduce the patient's morbidity and mortality.

TAKE HOME MESSAGES

- Neural antibodies are defined as antibodies that are targeted against neural antigens and produce neuronal injury which may be due to T-cell mediated or antibody-mediated mechanisms
- Basically, these are classified into physiological (to clear protein aggregates) and pathological origin and these pathological antibodies are further classified into malignancy associated and nonmalignancy associated
- The antibodies against cell surface antigens are predominantly nonparaneoplastic, whereas antibodies against nuclear/cytosolic antigens are predominantly of paraneoplastic origin
- Neuronal injury in the presence of these neural antibodies results from multiple effector mechanisms (IgG mediated in nonparaneoplastic setting or T-cell mediated in paraneoplastic setting)
- The nuclear/cytosolic antibodies are not directly involved in pathogenesis of the disease but the neuronal damage is mediated by T-cell mechanism
- Cell surface and synaptic antibodies result in disruption in the function of target antigen, thereby leading to neuronal dysfunction
- These neuronal antibodies produce characteristic syndromes in paraneoplastic and nonparaneoplastic setting which includes autoimmune encephalitis, autoimmune epilepsy, autoimmune myelopathies, autoimmune movement disorders, autoimmune cerebellopathies and others
- Autoimmune epilepsy should be suspected in those patients who present with new onset status epilepticus, refractory status epilepticus, rapid cognitive decline and early age of onset
- Treatment for antibodies associated with paraneoplastic is mainly focused towards neoplasm
- Immunotherapy is the mainstay of treatment for nonparaneoplastic autoimmune syndromes like NMO spectrum disorder, autoimmune epilepsy, autoimmune encephalitis and others.

SUGGESTED READINGS

1. Conrad K1, Roggenbuck D, Reinhold D, et al. Autoantibody diagnostics in clinical practice. Autoimmun Rev. 2012;11(3):207-11.
2. Darnell RB, Posner JB. Paraneoplastic syndromes involving the nervous system. N Engl J Med. 2003;349(16):1543-54.
3. Gold M, Pul R, Bach JP, et al. Pathogenic and physiological autoantibodies in the central nervous system. Immunol Rev. 2012;248:68-86.
4. Hinson SR, Pittock SJ, Lucchinetti CF, et al. Pathogenic potential of IgG binding to water channel extracellular domain in neuromyelitis optica. Neurology. 2007;69(24):2221-31.
5. Iorio R, Lennon VA. Neural antigen-specific autoimmune disorders. Immunol Rev. 2012;248(1):104-21.
6. Lancaster E, Dalmau J. Neuronal autoantigens--pathogenesis, associated disorders and antibody testing. Nat Rev Neurol. 2012;8(7):380-90.
7. McKeon A, Pittock SJ. Paraneoplastic encephalomyelopathies: Pathology and mechanisms. Acta Neuropathol. 2011;122(4):381-400.

8. Middeldorp J, Hol EM. GFAP in health and disease. Prog Neurobiol. 2011;93:421-43.
9. Papadopoulos MC, Verkman AS. Aquaporin 4 and neuromyelitis optica. Lancet Neurol. 2012;11:535-44.
10. Pekny M, Pekna M. Astrocyte intermediate filaments in CNS pathologies and regeneration. J Pathol. 2004;204:428-37.
11. Pittock SJ, Kryzer TJ, Lennon VA. Paraneoplastic antibodies coexist and predict cancer, not neurological syndrome. Ann Neurol. 2004;56(5):715-9.
12. Pittock SJ, Lennon VA, McKeon A, et al. Eculizumab in AQP4-IgG-positive relapsing neuromyelitis optica spectrum disorders: an open-label pilot study. Lancet Neurol. 2013;12(6):554-62.
13. Pittock SJ, Palace J. Paraneoplastic and idiopathic autoimmune neurologic disorders: Approach to diagnosis and treatment. Handb Clin Neurol. 2016;133:165-83.
14. Plonquet A, Gherardi RK, Créange A, et al. Oligoclonal T-cells in blood and target tissues of patients with anti-Hu syndrome. J Neuroimmunol. 2002;122(1-2):100-5.
15. Posner JB. Neurologic complications of cancer. Philadelphia, PA: FA Davis Company; 1995. pp. 353-84.
16. Quek AM, Britton JW, McKeon A, et al. Autoimmune epilepsy: Clinical characteristics and response to immunotherapy. Arch Neurol. 2012;69(5):582-93.
17. Rash JE, Yasumura T, Hudson CS, et al. Direct immunogold labeling of aquaporin-4 in square arrays of astrocyte and ependymocyte plasma membranes in rat brain and spinal cord. Proc Natl Acad Sci USA. 1998;95:11981-6.
18. Tobin WO, Pittock SJ. Autoimmune neurology of the central nervous system. Continuum (Minneap Minn). 2017;23(3, Neurology of Systemic Disease):627-53.
19. Waters P, Pettingill P, Lang B. Detection methods for neural autoantibodies. Handb Clin Neurol. 2016;133:147-63.

CHAPTER 3

Laboratory Evaluation of Neuronal Antibodies

Annamma Mathai, Davidson Devasia, Parvathy Rajan, Sudheeran Kannoth

INTRODUCTION

Autoimmune neurology is called as the 21st century subspecialty of neurology. Being an etiology based subspecialty, it transects all other traditional subspecialties of neurology like cognition, movement disorder, epilepsy, sleep, autonomic disorders, and so on. Apart from the neurological subspecialties, it also closely interacts with other medical/surgical specialties [e.g., gynecology in N-methyl-D-aspartic acid (NMDA) receptor encephalitis for management of teratoma, oncology in case of paraneoplastic neurological syndromes, gastroenterology in cases of hiccoughs in neuromyelitis optica spectrum disorder and gastroparesis with dysautonomia, and psychiatry in cases of autoimmune encephalitis]. Laboratory evaluation for neuronal antibodies are very important in the diagnosis of autoimmune neurological syndromes.

HISTORY

First neuronal antibody was recognized in 1976—Purkinje cell cytoplasmic antibody (PCA) Trotter (Tr). This was identified with indirect immunofluorescence (IIF). Subsequently PCA-1 (anti-Yo) was described in 1983 again by IIF. Subsequently, more and more antibodies were described and the list is ever expanding.

INDICATIONS FOR TESTING OF NEURONAL ANTIBODIES

Autoimmune neurological diseases can present with a wide variety of manifestations. Some of the presentations can be called as signature disease where you can identify them by clinical/radiological means. For example, limbic encephalitis (clinical and radiological), paraneoplastic myelitis (radiological), chorea in elderly [collapsin response mediator protein-5 antibody (CRMP5) mediated], encephalomyelitis, NMDA receptor encephalitis (psychosis with movement disorder, seizures), faciobrachial dystonic seizure [leucine-rich glioma-inactivated 1 (LGI1) antibody mediated], neuromyelits optica spectrum disorder (aquaporin-4 antibody). In these scenarios, the indication for neuronal antibody testing is very evident. However, the situation may be different in other cases. In other cases, multi-axial neurological involvement (different parts of central and peripheral nervous system), presence of risk factors like personal/family history of autoimmunity (rheumatoid arthritis, hypothyroidism, pernicious anemia, vitiligo, systemic lupus erythematosus, dermatological conditions like psoriasis, lichen planus and pemphigus, myasthenia gravis, etc.), and malignancy (paraneoplastic) are strong pointers for an autoimmune etiology in the given neurological disorder. Presence of stigmata of autoimmunity/malignancy in the history or examination (like polyarthralgia/arthritis, deformity, rash, cachexia, bone pains, unexplained weight loss, and smoking) also should be considered as pointer towards autoimmunity as the etiology in the given case. Preliminary laboratory investigations like elevated erythrocyte sedimentation rate, C-reactive protein, presence of nonorgan specific autoimmune markers like antinuclear antibody, rheumatoid factor all are good clues for an underlying autoimmune etiology in neurological disorder. Apart from this, in all unexplained neurological diseases, we should suspect autoimmune etiology and investigate with neuronal antibody testing.

SAMPLES FOR TESTING

Wherever possible, do the testing on paired sample—serum and cerebrospinal fluid (CSF). N-methyl-D-aspartic acid receptor antibody has a better yield in CSF (100%) than serum (85.6%). For other antibodies, serum has a better yield. However, occasionally when serum did not yield the antibody, CSF may become positive as in neuromyelitis optica (NMO) IgG.

TRANSPORTATION OF SAMPLES

Blood samples to be collected in vacutainers for testing serum. Serum separator tubes (yellow cap) are the best and if not available can be collected on red capped vacutainers. Cerebrospinal fluid is to be collected on white capped tube which contains no anticoagulant. Screw capped containers are important, especially if the sample is to be transported to the laboratory at a far-away location. Antibodies are stable at room temperature up to 72 hours. If it is expected that the transport will take more than 72 hours, samples to be packed and sent with ice pack/cooling gel/dry ice. Eppendorf tubes are good for transportation of samples as they are leak proof.

CLASSIFICATION OF ANTIBODIES

Antibodies can be classified as paraneoplastic and nonparaneoplastic based on cancer association. Paraneoplastic antibodies are cancer associated antibodies and are markers of malignancy and in the right clinical context indicate that the given neurological syndrome is paraneoplastic. The disease here is not antibody mediated but T-cell mediated and has a poorer prognosis. Nonparaneoplastic antibodies are classified as cell surface antibodies and many of them are antibody mediated and have a better prognosis. Sometimes same antibody can be paraneopalstic as well as nonparaneoplastic (e.g., NMDA receptor antibody is mostly nonparaneopalstic but can be paraneoplastic associated with teratoma). Based on the location of target molecule, they can be classified as intracellular and cell surface antibodies.

NOMENCLATURE OF ANTIBODIES

The first antibody was named after the doctor who discovered it—PCA Tr (Tr stands for Trotter, PCA for Purkinje cell cytoplasmic antibody). Subsequent antibodies were described with the first two letters of the name of the index patients from whom the antibodies were detected for the first time. Anti-Yo (patient's name Young), anti-Hu (patient's name Hull), and anti-Ma (patient's name Margret). Subsequently, another nomenclature also was developed based on the staining pattern on IIF of tissue—antineuronal nuclear antibody (ANNA), PCA, antiglial nuclear antibody (AGNA). Anti-Hu is ANNA-1, anti-Ri is ANNA-2, and anti-Yo is PCA-1 as per this nomenclature.

Later on, newer antibodies were named after their target antigenic molecule—CRMP5, amphiphysin, and NMDA receptor antibody.

METHODS OF TESTING

Different methods of testing are available ranging from the conventional IIF testing on tissue sections to live cell-based assay. Indirect immunofluorescence on tissue section is one of the best options as initial screening test. Its advantages are that it is the most time tested and cost-effective test and enables to discover a large number of antigens including the new unnamed/uncharacterized ones. It helps in detecting multiple antibodies at a time. Once antibodies are detected by IIF on tissue sections, it is to be confirmed with another method like western blot/line blot. This is the standard practice followed in major international reference neuroimmunology laboratories like Mayo Clinic and Oxford University. Another method available is enzyme-linked immunosorbent assay. Its main limitation is its inability to detect the cell surface antibodies like NMDA and LGI1, where antigenicity is based on conformational property of the protein. Indirect immunofluorescence on cell-based assays are better option in this situation. There are other methods like flow cytometry and immunofluorescence on live cells.

Doing the whole panel of the antibody is the best method as many a time more than one antibody can present with similar clinical features. For example, limbic encephalitis can be the presentation of LGI1 antibody, contactin associated protein-like 2 (CASPR2) antibody, ANNA-1antibody, and many other antibodies.

Please refer to chapter 2 for the list of antibodies, their cancer association, clinical manifestation, and whether they are directed to cell surface antigen or intracellular antigen.

INTERPRETATION OF THE TEST REPORTS

Like other laboratory investigations, neuronal antibodies test reports also to be interpreted carefully with reference to the clinical scenario. Paraneoplastic antibodies can be seen in cancer even without paraneoplastic syndrome; e.g. ANNA-1 antibody was seen in up to 16% of small cell cancer patients without neurological syndrome. So detection of paraneoplastic antibody should prompt them to search for the underlying malignancy. If one gets a cancer on further investigation which is not predicted by the antibody, one should treat that cancer and continue searching for the cancer which is predicted by the antibody. Sometimes, the panel testing may yield more than one antibody and this can help to identify the malignancy. For example, if the patient tested positive for CRMP-5 antibody along with acetyl choline receptor antibody and anti-striational muscle antibody, it indicates underlying thymoma. Amphiphysin antibody alone in a woman suggests a breast malignancy while amphiphysin with ANNA-1 or CRMP-5 antibodies points towards a lung malignancy. In Lambert-Eaton myasthenic syndrome (LEMS), voltage gated calcium channel antibody for P/Q and N are positive. If AGNA-1 also is positive, it tells that it is a paraneopalstic LEMS.

In case of nonparaneoplastic antibodies, a positive CSF NMDA antibody in the presence of symptoms in one of the six clinical domains is sufficient to make the definitive diagnosis of NMDA receptor encephalitis.

A positive antibody indicates the presence of an immune reaction against the particular antigen. Hence, interpretation of test positivity should be done carefully in the clinical context. Presence of antibody in CSF will be stronger evidence. Always there is a need to rule out alternative diagnosis as in some cases the symptoms are not caused by the antibody. As already mentioned with paraneoplastic antibody, in a patient with malignancy and encephalopathy secondary to septic/metabolic/nutritional cause, the presence of the antibody is only a marker of immunological response to cancer. Contactin-associated protein-like 2 antibody in CSF shows a greater propensity for encephalitis while in serum alone it favors a peripheral nervous system presentation (neuromyotonia). If you get a PCA-1 (anti-Yo) antibody positive in male patient, you have to cross-check it as it is extremely rare in men (<20 cases reported in men).

What to Do if You Get Negative Reports?

A negative result on a strongly suspected case should prompt us to do follow-up testing. If only one sample, serum or CSF is tested and it is negative, testing of the other sample, i.e., CSF if serum was negative and serum if CSF was negative is the next step. If both are negative, retesting at a later date is required. Testing for the whole panel of antibody is another solution. As clinical phenotypes can look alike for different antibodies, a less experienced physician may think that the longitudinally extensive transverse myelitis is caused by NMO IgG but it may be due to myelin oligodendrocyte glycoprotein IgG. A stiff person syndrome may be caused by GAD65, amphiphysin, or glycine antibody. Cerebellar ataxia patient tested for PCA-1 (anti-Yo) may be negative but if whole panel is tested voltage gated calcium channel antibody would have come positive. A negative test does not exclude the diagnosis as antibodies are not the sole criteria for diagnosis. For example, the diagnosis of NMDA receptor encephalitis can be made even in the absence of antibodies if the clinical and other laboratory criteria are met (probable NMDA receptor encephalitis). In the meantime, antibodies, if positive in a classical syndrome, is diagnostic. Similarly, diagnosis of NMO spectrum disorders can be made even if antibodies were negative. Antibodies are positive only in 60–70% cases of paraneoplastic syndromes. Even if antibodies are negative, the diagnosis can be made based on the proposed criteria, if cancer is detected and neurological condition improves with cancer removal. Up to 22% cases with positive onconeural antibodies, no cancer is detected with regular imaging techniques and in some cases cancers were not picked even at autopsy. This is presumed to be due to small foci of malignancy and strong immune response against it.

CONCLUSION

Laboratory evaluation for neuronal antibodies is a very important tool in the diagnosis of suspected autoimmune neurological syndrome. A good clinical and laboratory correlation is the most important step in making the diagnosis. As newer and newer antibodies are being described, it is important to have testing done in dedicated laboratories with clinicians trained in autoimmune neurology for better results as well as interpretation of results in the clinical context.

TAKE HOME MESSAGES

- Neuronal antibody evaluation is an important tool in diagnosis of suspected autoimmune neurological syndromes
- Testing with both serum and CSF sample should be performed wherever possible
- Evaluation with panel of antibodies is more appropriate than ordering a single antibody as many phenotypically similar syndromes are caused by/associated with different antibodies
- Negative test does not exclude the diagnosis
- History and family history of autoimmune disease, family history of cancer, clinical signs suggestive of autoimmunity on examination are the clues for initiating neuronal antibody evaluation
- Good clinical and laboratory correlation is very essential in arriving at diagnosis
- As newer and newer antibodies are being described, it is important to have testing done in dedicated laboratories with clinicians trained in autoimmune neurology for better results as well as interpretation of results in the clinical context.

SUGGESTED READINGS

1. Graus F, Titulaer MJ, Balu R, et al. A clinical approach to diagnosis of autoimmune encephalitis. Lancet Neurol. 2016;15(4):391-404.
2. Gresa-Arribas N, Titulaer MJ, Torrents A, et al. Diagnosis and significance of antibody titers in anti-NMDA receptor encephalitis, a retrospective study. Lancet Neurol. 2014;13(2):167.
3. Horta ES, Lennon VA, Lachance DH, et al. Neural autoantibody clusters aid diagnosis of cancer. Clin Can Res. 2014;20(14):3862-9.
4. Joubert B, Saint-Martin M, Noraz N, et al. Characterization of a subtype of autoimmune encephalitis with anti-contactin-associated protein-like 2 antibodies in the cerebrospinal fluid, prominent limbic symptoms, and seizures. JAMA Neurol. 2016;73(9):1115-24.
5. Kannoth S. Paraneoplastic neurologic syndrome: A practical approach. Ann Indian Acad Neurol. 2012;15(1):6.
6. Lennon VA. Paraneoplastic autoantibodies: The case for a descriptive generic nomenclature. Neurology. 1994;44(12):2236-40.
7. McKeon A, Pittock SJ, Lennon VA. CSF complements serum for evaluating paraneoplastic antibodies and NMO-IgG. Neurology. 2011;76(12):1108-10.
8. Sabater L, Titulaer M, Saiz A, et al. SOX1 antibodies are markers of paraneoplastic Lambert–Eaton myasthenic syndrome. Neurology. 2008;70(12):924-8.

CHAPTER 4

Autoimmune Dementia

Lakshmi Narasimhan Ranganathan, Arun Shivaraman Mulanur Murugesan, Lenin Sankar Palanisamy, Sreenivas Umaiorubahan Meenakshisundaram, Kannan Vangiliappan, Guhan Ramamurthy, Srinivasan Avathvadi Venkatesan

INTRODUCTION

Dementia significantly impairs activities of daily living in the affected patients. It is increasing in prevalence owing to the increasing longevity resulting from improving healthcare. Screening patients with dementia for secondary causes of dementia is a preferred prerequisite. The role of autoimmunity in the causation of dementia has been overwhelming and revealing; and its treatment has advanced and improved the quality of life of affected patients. The entity of autoimmune dementia, the pathogenesis, and its management has broadened since discovery. The contribution of autoimmunity has scaled up from the autoimmune dementia to cognitive decline secondary to systemic autoimmune diseases. Further, recent studies have suggested the contribution of autoimmunity in the causation of primary dementia. In this chapter, we discuss the multifaceted autoimmune processes targeting cognition under the following headings:
- Autoimmune dementia
- Systemic autoimmunity and dementia
- Role of autoimmunity in primary dementia.

Classification of Autoimmune Dementia

The autoimmune dementia can be classified as intracellular or extracellular based on the pathogenesis. In autoimmune dementia with intracellular antigen, the antibody is not pathological and serves as a marker of the disease. The disease process is mediated through T-cell mediated process or unidentified antibody. In extracellular pathogenesis, the antibody binds to the target antigen and causes disease process through competitive blockade of receptors, internalization of receptors and antibody-mediated cell-dependent cytotoxicity. Hence, intracellular autoimmune dementia responds poorly to immunotherapy as compared to extracellular autoimmune dementia (Flowchart 1).

Extracellular Autoimmune Dementia

The various extracellular autoimmune dementias are discussed as follows:
- *Anti-voltage gated potassium channel (VGKC) antibody*: VGKC is located in the plasma membrane in both central and peripheral nervous system. It is involved in repolarization of the neurons. The antibodies are directed against the associated proteins of these channels—leucine-rich glioma-inactivated-1 (LGI1) protein and contactin-associated protein-like 2 (CASPR2). Adult population (50–70 years) is usually affected.

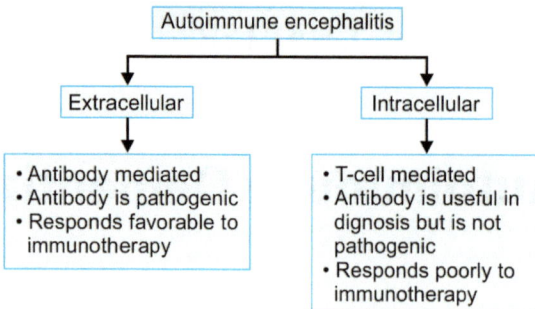

FLOWCHART 1: The differences between intracellular and extracellular autoimmune encephalitis.

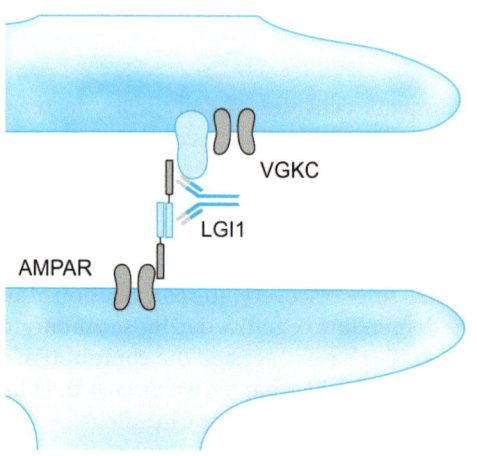

AMPAR, alpha-amino-3-hydroxy-5-methyl-4-isoxazolepropionic acid receptor; LGI1, leucine-rich glioma-inactivated-1.

FIG. 1: Voltage-gated potassium channel (VGKC) and associated proteins located at synapse in central nervous system.

Leucine-rich glioma-inactivated-1 is a synaptic protein that interacts with potassium channel (Kv1 subunit) and is essential for the localization of the potassium channel (Fig. 1). Antibodies against these proteins lead to defective functioning of the potassium channel resulting in clinical symptoms. Leucine-rich glioma-inactivated-1 is located in the central nervous system (CNS). Patients can have seizures (generalized tonic-clonic seizures, faciobrachial dystonic seizures or partial seizures), cognitive dysfunction (disorientation and executive dysfunction), behavioral symptoms and insomnia. Some patients may have hyponatremia. These antibodies are seen in both cerebrospinal fluid (CSF) and serum. Serum assay has better sensitivity (100%) than CSF assay (88%). Magnetic resonance imaging (MRI) brain reveals temporal lobe T2/fluid-attenuated inversion recovery (FLAIR) hyperintensity.

Contactin-associated protein-like 2 is a membranal adhesion protein which helps in clustering of the potassium channel in the juxtaparanodal region of the nerve terminal and thus regulates the action potential depolarization (Fig. 2). These channels are seen both in central and peripheral nervous system. Patients may have

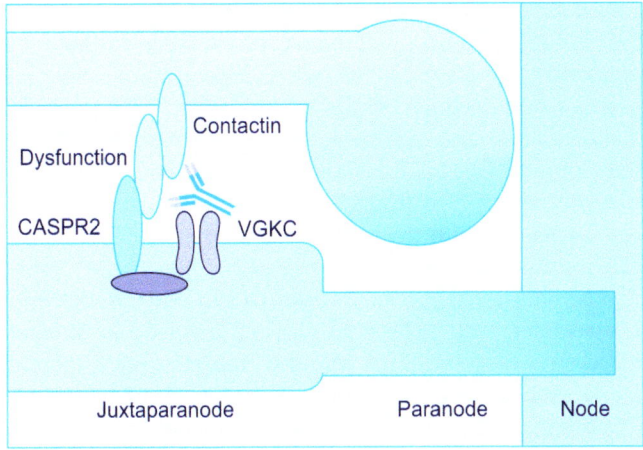

FIG. 2: Juxtaparanodal regions showing voltage-gated potassium channel (VGKC) complex with associated proteins. Antibody binds to the contactin-associated protein-like 2 (CASPR2) protein.

involvement of peripheral nervous system resulting in Morvan's syndrome (peripheral nerve hyperexcitability), characteristically has myokymia and muscle cramps. Central nervous system involvement results in cognitive decline, dysautonomia and sleep disturbances. Serum antibody levels are more sensitive than CSF levels. MRI brain may be normal or reveal temporal lobe hyperintensity. Contactin-associated protein-like 2 antibodies may be seen in thymoma patients.

Antibodies mediated directly against the potassium channel (anti-VGKC) have been documented. These patients have positive anti-VGKC antibody but negative for LGI1 and CASPR2 antibodies. Clinical manifestations may be any of the above-mentioned features. These antibodies may also present as frontotemporal dementia and may mimic Creutzfeldt–Jakob disease. The wide clinical presentation may suggest that the target of these antibodies may yet be unidentified.

These antibodies can be paraneoplastic [breast, small cell lung cancer (SCLC), thymoma and prostate] or nonparaneoplastic. Patients having these antibodies respond well to immunotherapy

- *NMDAR (N-methyl-D-aspartate receptor) antibody*: NMDAR is a transmembrane protein which can bind to both, glycine (NR1 subunit) and glutamate (NR2 subunit) and mediate membrane signaling. Antibodies against NMDAR are directed against NR1 subunit. These antibodies are commonly seen in young females. Clinical features include behavioral and psychiatric disturbances (80%), seizures (70%), orofacial dyskinesia and other movement disorders, cognitive decline with speech and language disturbances, and autonomic disturbances. Some patients may develop central hypoventilation. Anti-NMDAR antibodies are seen in both serum and CSF. MRI brain reveals abnormality in around 50% patients (hippocampal and basal ganglia T2/FLAIR hyperintensity). Electroencephalography (EEG) reveals a characteristic delta brush pattern. Anti-NMDAR antibodies are seen in ovarian teratoma. These patients respond well to immunotherapy
- *Alpha-amino-3-hydroxy-5-methyl-4-isoxazolepropionic acid (AMPA) receptor antibody*: AMPA receptors are membrane-bound receptors binding to glutamate. It is

involved in excitation and synaptic transmission in CNS. Antibody against these receptors results in loss of function of the receptors. These antibodies are commonly seen in females within age group of 40–60 years. Clinical manifestations include limbic encephalitis (cognitive decline, behavioral symptoms and confusion) cerebellar symptoms, hallucinations and hypersomnia. Seizures have also reported. MRI brain reveals mesial temporal T2/FLAIR hyperintensity. Antibodies are found both in CSF and serum. Alpha-amino-3-hydroxy-5-methyl-4-isoxazolepropionic acid receptor antibodies are associated with thymoma, and lung and breast carcinoma. Patients respond well to immunotherapy

- *Anti-dipeptidyl peptidase–like protein 6 (anti-DPPX) antibody*: DPPX is a regulatory glycoprotein associated with potassium channel involved in integration of neural signals and prevents the retrograde impulse transmission. Dipeptidyl peptidase–like protein 6 is seen in both central and peripheral nervous system. Antibodies against DPPX protein in CNS results in cognitive decline, seizures, agitation, tremors, hallucinations and confusion. Progressive encephalomyelitis with rigidity and myoclonus (PERM) is a well-described entity seen with anti-DPPX antibody syndrome. Anti-DPPX antibody affecting the enteric nervous system causes the gastrointestinal dysmotility syndrome. Antibodies are present in both serum and CSF. MRI brain may be normal, diffuse white matter T2/FLAIR hyperintensity or focal temporal T2/FLAIR hyperintensity. Electroencephalography may show diffuse or focal slowing. These are associated with B-cell neoplasms. They respond well to immunotherapy
- *Other antibodies*: Other antibodies have also been demonstrated sporadically in demented patients with underlying malignancy. They include antiglycine receptor antibodies in patients with thymoma and B-cell tumors manifesting as progressive encephalomyelitis with rigidity and myoclonus. Antiganglionic acetylcholine receptor antibody is seen in patients with adenocarcinoma of various organs and renal cell carcinoma. They can manifest with cognitive decline, encephalopathy, peripheral neuropathy and dysautonomia. Anti-gamma amino butyric acid (GABA)-B receptor antibodies may be seen in patients with small cell carcinoma lung manifesting as limbic encephalitis, seizures, or peripheral neuropathy.

Intracellular Autoimmune Dementia

Intracellular antibody-associated autoimmune dementias were described years before the extracellular antibody-associated autoimmune dementias. The characteristic features of intracellular antibody-associated dementias are:
- Intracellular antibody-associated dementias are much less common than the extracellular antibody-associated dementias
- They are almost always associated with neoplasms, whereas the extracellular antibody-associated autoimmune dementias are rarely associated with neoplasia
- They respond poorly to immunotherapy in contrast to extracellular antibody-associated dementias
- They respond to the treatment of the underlying malignancy in most cases even though not in all and the response may not be much rewarding as in extracellular antibody-associated dementias
- The clinical manifestations can be explained by the antigenic targets in case of extracellular antibody-associated autoimmune dementia, whereas it is not true in intracellular antibody-associated dementias

- The antibodies in the intracellular antibody associated dementias are not directly pathogenic and the main pathogenic mechanism is cytotoxic T-cell mediated neuronal death; and for the same reason, in most patients, the treatment may only halt the progression and may not revert the damage that has already occurred
- They often show positivity for multiple autoantibodies, hence a panel of paraneoplastic antibodies are to be requested if intracellular antibody-associated dementia is suspected and the significance of the antibody titer has to be interpreted in the light of the patient's clinical manifestations
- Even though they are almost always paraneoplastic, neurological syndrome precedes the cancer diagnosis in most of them despite thorough investigation. Hence, European Federation of Neurological Sciences recommends cancer screening at 6-monthly interval for 4 years after the initial diagnosis of the neurological syndrome.

The various intracellular antibodies associated with dementias are:
- Anti-Hu or ANNA1 (antineuronal nuclear antibody 1)
- Anti-CRMP 5 (collapsin response mediator protein 5) or CV2
- Anti-Ma/Ta
- Anti-GAD (glutamic acid decarboxylase)
- Anti-AGNA/SOX-1 (anti-glial nuclear antibody)
- Anti-ANNA3 (antineuronal nuclear antibody 3)
- Anti-PCA (Purkinje cell cytoplasmic antibody type 2).

Anti-Hu or Antineuronal Nuclear Antibody 1-associated Dementia

Most commonly associated with SCLC. As many of 20% of patients with SCLC will show anti-Hu antibody positivity, whereas only less than 1% of patients with SCLC develop clinical manifestations. It is more commonly seen in males. Apart from the cognitive and behavioral manifestations, others include neuropathy, cerebellar ataxia and dysautonomia. There are no specific neuroimaging features that help in the diagnosis. Cerebrospinal fluid analysis will be abnormal in at least 70% of patients but is nonspecific and includes elevated protein, elevated immunoglobulin (Ig) G index and lymphocytic pleocytosis. In approximately 70% of the patients with anti-Hu antibody-associated dementia, the neurological manifestations precede the diagnosis of the underlying malignancy. Hence, periodic screening for the malignancy in question is mandatory. Treatment of the underlying malignancy with or without immunotherapy has shown significant difference in terms of clinical outcome when compared to treatment with immunotherapy alone.

Anti-collapsin Response Mediator Protein 5-associated Dementia

The CRMP is involved in neurogenesis. These antibodies are associated with SCLC more commonly and with thymoma less commonly. Both men and women are equally affected. The various neurological manifestations associated with anti-CRMP5 antibodies are cerebellar syndrome, various movement disorders including chorea, seizures, cranial and peripheral neuropathy, and cognitive and behavioral disturbances. Cerebrospinal fluid analysis will be abnormal but nonspecific as in case of other intracellular antibody-associated dementias. MRI of brain features T2/FLAIR hyperintense patches which may or may not be contrast enhancing. Treatment of the underlying malignancy shows drastic improvement, although there are anecdotal reports of symptomatic improvement with immunotherapy. As almost all of them are associated with malignancy, periodic screening is essential as in other intracellular antibody-associated dementia if the initial evaluation is negative for malignancy.

Anti Ma/Ta Antibody-associated Dementia

The cellular function of Ma protein is speculated to be transcription of ribonucleic acid. Isolated anti-Ma2 antibody positivity is seen with germ-cell tumor of testis; hence, it has a male preponderance. The neurological manifestations include peripheral neuropathy and brainstem syndromes in addition to the cognitive and behavioral symptoms. Neuroimaging with MRI may show nonspecific T2/FLAIR hyperintensities. The CSF shows nonspecific inflammatory features and it is observed in up to 50% of individuals. Treatment of the malignancy is associated with excellent neurological outcome in contrast to other intracellular antibody-associated dementias.

Unlike patients with isolated Ma2 antibody-associated dementia, patients who are positive for both Ma1 and Ma2 are predominantly females and the underlying malignancy may be any one of the following—colon, ovary, breast, and lymphoma. They may present with a broad range of cognitive symptoms and other structures involved in neuraxis include cerebellum, brainstem and autonomic nervous system. Nonspecific focal T2 hyperintense lesions with or without atrophy may be seen in MRI of brain. The CSF analysis will usually be inflammatory with elevated protein, lymphocytic pleocytosis and oligoclonal bands and, at times, CSF analysis may be totally normal. As with other intracellular antibody-associated dementias, the neurological syndrome precedes the neoplasm; hence, periodic screening for the malignancy is essential. Unlike isolated Ma2 antibody-associated dementia, these patients have a poor clinical outcome.

Anti-glutamic Acid Decarboxylase Antibody-associated Dementia

The cellular function of the enzyme GAD is GABA synthesis. Antibodies against GAD are also associated with stiff person syndrome, type 1 diabetes and also seen in a significant proportion of normal individuals. In contrary to other intracellular antibody-associated dementias, they are rarely paraneoplastic. The age at onset is typically young. In most of them, the initial presentation would be seizures of temporal lobe semiology and cognitive manifestations are observed late in the course. They are usually associated with other autoantibodies like thyroid peroxidase antibody and anti-parietal cell antibody. The CSF analysis will be in favor of an inflammatory pathology in most. T2/FLAIR hyperintensity associated with swelling will be observed in medial temporal lobes. Anti-GAD antibody titers are to be interpreted cautiously for the following reasons—the significant titers for diabetes and neurological syndrome varies, a positive anti-GAD antibody in low titers are common, and a low titer in the absence of typical clinical manifestations are not clinically relevant. Even though anti-GAD antibody-associated dementias are rarely paraneoplastic, they are poorly responsive to immunotherapy. The seizures associated with them are much more difficult to be managed than those associated with anti-NMDAR encephalitis. Recently described intracellular antibody-associated syndromes:

Anti-glial Nuclear Antibody-associated Dementia

Anti-glial nuclear antibody is known to be associated with paraneoplastic cerebellar degeneration and Lambert-Eaton myasthenic syndrome and they are also useful in predicting the risk of developing SCLC in patients with Lambert-Eaton myasthenic syndrome. Recently, there are few case reports of limbic encephalitis and associated cognitive dysfunction in patients who are positive for AGNA antibody. The intracellular target of AGNA antibody is SOX-1, a transcription factor involved in neural development.

Antineuronal Nuclear Antibody 3-associated Dementia

The most commonly associated neurological manifestations include brain stem encephalitis, sensory neuropathy, motor neuropathy, cerebellar ataxia and myelopathy. There are anecdotal reports of limbic encephalitis and associated dementia in patients with ANNA-3. Their most common association is with SCLC.

Anti-Purkinje Cell Cytoplasmic Antibody Type 2-associated Dementia

They have a strong association with SCLC. Apart from dementia, other neuraxial structures that were involved in these patients are brainstem, neuromuscular junction, peripheral nerves, cerebellum and autonomic nervous system.

Systemic Autoimmunity in Dementia

Patients with systemic autoimmune conditions can also develop dementia. Common autoimmune conditions that may manifest as dementia include:
- Systemic lupus erythematosus (SLE)
- Rheumatoid arthritis
- Sjogren's syndrome
- Celiac disease
- Ulcerative colitis
- Goodpasture syndrome
- Sarcoidosis
- Behçet's disease
- Autoimmune dementia
- Addison's disease
- Psoriasis
- Type 1 diabetes.

Autoimmune disorder increases the likelihood of developing dementia by 20%. The risk for Alzheimer's disease (AD) and vascular dementia were also higher. The increased risk for vascular dementia is possibly due to the association between autoimmune diseases and accelerated atherosclerosis that also predisposes to cardiovascular and cerebrovascular diseases in these patients. Cognitive decline in SLE is often temporary. Around 90% of SLE patients develop neuropsychiatric symptoms. Cognitive impairment (80%) and mood disorder (43%) are very common. Cognitive decline in executive function, attention, planning and working memory was often noticed in neuropsychiatric SLE. Increased risk of dementia in SLE patient is determined by multiple factors like the disease process, increased prevalence of cardiovascular risk factors and treatment. Executive function and processing speed were more affected in SLE patients who tested positive for anti-cardiolipin autoantibody. These patients also develop recurrent cerebral microischemia and stroke which results in increased risk of dementia. Corticosteroid usage in SLE impairs attention, executive function and memory.

Systemic lupus erythematosus also causes changes in the neuroanatomical structure. Cerebral atrophy, periventricular white-matter changes, hemorrhage and infarction were commonly noticed in MRI brain of patients with SLE. Volumetric analysis in SLE patients showed volume loss in the hippocampus, corpus callosum, cerebral cortex, and cerebellum (Fig. 3).

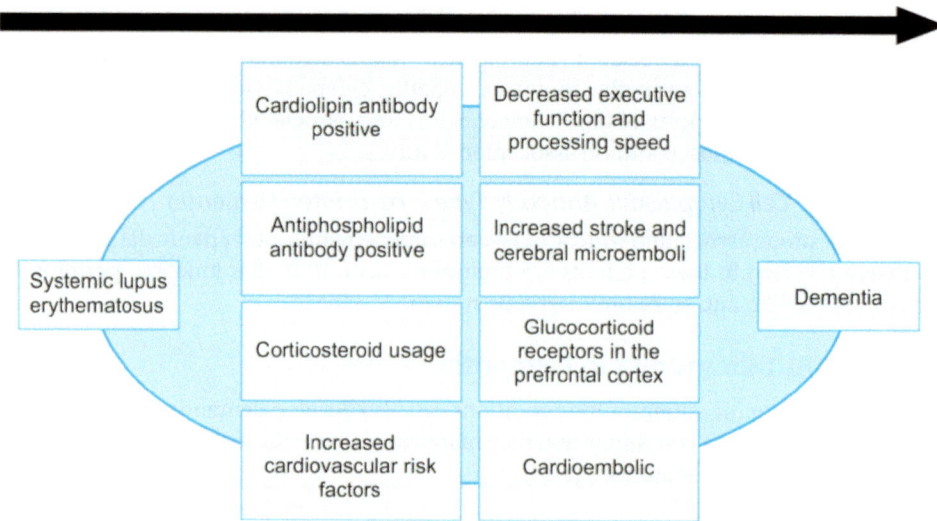

FIG. 3: Various mechanism of dementia in systemic lupus erythematosus.

Two different opinions prevail regarding association between rheumatoid arthritis and AD.
1. Patients with rheumatoid arthritis were found to be protective against AD. This was attributed to the reason that nonsteroidal anti-inflammatory drugs (NSAIDs) like aspirin and paracetamol intake have been associated with reduced risk of AD
2. Arthritis itself in addition to NSAIDs usage had a protective role against developing AD. One study showed 13% increased risk of developing dementia in patients having rheumatoid arthritis.

When compared to people without diabetes, older people with type 1 diabetes had 80% higher risk for developing dementia. Only a fewer studies have been conducted on the risk of developing dementia in type 1 diabetes. This is due to the increased longevity of patients with type 1 diabetes, long enough to be at a risk of cognitive dysfunction. Possible mechanisms that may lead to dementia in type 1 diabetes were hypoglycemic episodes, microvascular risk factors and depression.

Sjogren's syndrome in association with vasculitis and meningoencephalitis has been reported. Dementia and subtle cognitive decline have been noticed in patients with Sjogren's syndrome. Psoriasis was associated with 29% excess risk of developing dementia. Crohn's disease had 10% increased risk of developing dementia on subsequent follow-up. In patients with polyarteritis nodosa, dementia may manifest after peripheral involvement during the course of the disease. Patients with sarcoidosis who develop diffuse meningoencephalitis may develop dementia. In Behcet's disease, sometimes the behavior changes may be the first symptom followed by difficulty in information processing, memory and executive functioning.

Role of Autoimmunity in Primary Dementia

The primary dementias are believed to be idiopathic with genetic and environmental influences. Recent evidence has emerged that some of these neurodegenerative disorders might also have a component of autoimmunity and inflammation associated with them.

Of the primary dementias, AD and frontotemporal lobar degeneration (FTLD) have been shown to have a higher association of autoimmunity.

Alzheimer's Disease

Alzheimer's disease is characterized by a chronic degenerative process with accumulation of amyloid-beta (Aβ) plaques in the cerebral cortex. Evidence has emerged that these plaques are stimuli for the activation of inflammatory responses via, microglia and has been shown to produce neuronal damage. However, labelling studies using benzodiazepines have not shown a consistently elevated microglial signal at sites of Aβ plaques. This has been postulated to be due to a possibility of benzodiazepines binding preferentially to microglia not involved in interactions with the plaques.

Other findings supporting an autoimmune component of AD include the high concentration of Monocyte chemoattractant protein 1 in plaques, which may lead to accumulation of reactive astrocytes. These reactive astrocytes induce neural proliferation leading to dystrophic neuron formation. Astrocytes have also been shown to increase activation of nuclear factor-κB (NF-κB) and CCAAT/enhancer binding protein delta (CEBPδ) on exposure to AD plaques. These factors fuel the inflammatory cascade and lead to further neuronal damage. Calcineurin has also been shown to be increased in reactive astrocytes in AD. This is another factor which leads to a proinflammatory state.

Complement activation via the classical pathway has been demonstrated *in vitro* by Aβ plaques. Central nervous system specific antibodies have also been demonstrated to be elevated in the CSF of patients with AD. These Igs have been found to be deposited in the amyloid plaques. These Igs are found in normal patients as well. However, neurodegeneration was found to be significantly more common among Ig-positive neurons compared to Ig-negative neurons. These Ig are proposed to cause cell death by activation of caspase-3. Dysfunction of the blood–brain barrier has been proposed as the cause for permeation of the autoantibodies into the CNS.

Other evidence for an inflammatory basis of AD arises from the protective effects of NSAIDs on the accumulation of Aβ plaques. Epidemiological data suggests that long-term NSAID use is associated with a decreased risk and delayed onset of AD.

Autoantibodies to adenosine triphosphate (ATP) synthase have been shown to be pathogenic. They inhibit ATP synthesis leading to mitochondrial dysfunction and cell death. The intraventricular administration of these antibodies in mice has shown to produce cognitive decline and hippocampal atrophy. Ceramide antibodies have also been implicated in increasing the amyloid plaque burden.

Frontotemporal Degeneration

Among the many variants of FTLD, the TDP43 related subtypes semantic variant primary progressive aphasia and deficiency in progranulin (PGRN) have been shown not to be associated with higher rates of inflammation. Increased levels of tumor necrosis factor (TNF)-α have been found in these patients compared to controls. Both these subtypes are proposed to have a similar neuropathology which occurs as a result of elevated TNF-α and the resultant inflammation leading to FTLD-TDP type C neuropathology.

Further evidence is obtained from recent studies showing that circulating anti-PGRN antibodies can decrease PGRN to levels comparable with those occurring in FTLD patients with granulin mutations—the causative agent in PGRN subtype. There has also been a case report of a patient with early onset FTLD having anti-AMPA antibodies GluR3 as an association. The link between systemic immunity and primary dementia has been mentioned earlier in this chapter.

Management

The epidemiological data suggesting a protective effect of NSAIDs on AD has led to multiple studies on the efficacy of these drugs as a treatment option for AD. However, clinical drug trials have not shown any clear-cut benefit supporting the use of NSAIDs in established disease. The protective effect needs to be explored in preclinical stages of AD and this still remains an area of no clarity.

The finding that natural antibodies to Aβ are protective against AD has led to exploration of passive immunization as a possible therapeutic option. Rarely, these antibodies have been found to cause cerebral amyloid angiopathy and may be pathogenic for AD in specific conditions.

Active immunization using Aβ vaccines and monoclonal Aβ antibodies has led to severe adverse effects and insignificant cognitive improvement. Recently, intravenous immunoglobulin (IVIG), which contains Aβ antibodies extracted from healthy individuals has led to improved cognitive function. More effective formulations of IVIG with catalytic antibodies to Aβ are under development, since this can lead to decreased risk of adverse effects. Aducanumab (BIIB037) is a natural antibody to Aβ fibrils. It has been shown to improve cognition and decrease plaque burden. Further studies are underway to confirm the efficacy and safety of this therapy.

Tau immunotherapy is another possibility under research in mice models. Tau specific monoclonal antibodies have been found to decrease tau as well as amyloid burden. The tau pathology has been associated with better correlation to cognitive impairment. Accordingly, this therapeutic option has shown signs of better cognitive improvement. All these options are under trial, and if approved would be a major step forward in the management of AD.

CONCLUSION

Autoimmunity has multifaceted mechanism leading to cognitive decline. It becomes essential to identify as it is a treatable cause. The identification and characterization of primary autoimmune dementia has been increasing at a fast pace. Early diagnosis and immunotherapy can produce drastic differences in the life of an individual. It provides treatment opportunities in primary dementia if its role is established. Further studies are required to study the role of immunotherapy in primary dementias.

TAKE HOME MESSAGES

- The incidence of autoimmune dementia is increasing. Recognition of this entity is important since treatment of the condition can reverse the dementia
- The autoimmune dementia may be primarily due to antibody targeted against neuronal antigen or as a part of systemic autoimmunity
- The primary autoimmune dementia is further classified as intracellular or extracellular based on the pathogenesis. This classification has treatment implications—extracellular autoimmune dementia responds favorably to immunotherapy while intracellular autoimmune dementia responds poorly to autoimmune dementia
- Systemic autoimmunity mediated dementia operates through multiple mechanisms
- Recent studies have suggested the role of autoimmunity in primary dementia. Further studies are required to affirm the findings.

SUGGESTED READINGS

1. Anderson AK, Phelps EA. Lesions of the human amygdala impair enhanced perception of emotionally salient events. Nature. 2001;411:305-9.
2. Appenzeller S, Bonilha L, Rio PA, et al. Longitudinal analysis of gray and white matter loss in patients with systemic lupus erythematosus. Neuroimage. 2007;34:694-701.
3. Appenzeller S, Rondina JM, Li LM, et al. Cerebral and corpus callosum atrophy in systemic lupus erythematosus. Arthritis Rheum. 2005;52:2783-9.
4. Biessels GJ, Staekenborg S, Brunner E, et al. Risk of dementia in diabetes mellitus: A systematic review. Lancet Neurol. 2006;5(1):64-74.
5. Blohorn A, Guegan-Massardier E, Triquenot A, et al. Antiphospholipid antibodies in the acute phase of cerebral ischaemia in young adults: A descriptive study of 139 patients. Cerebrovasc Dis. 2002;13:156-62.
6. Borroni B, Manes M, Alberici A, et al. Autoimmune frontotemporal dementia. Alzheimer Dis Assoc Disord. 2017;31(3):259-62.
7. Choi DW, Rothman SM. The role of glutamate neurotoxicity in hypoxic-ischemic neuronal death. Annu Rev Neurosci. 1990;13:171-82.
8. Ding H, Jian Z, Stary CM, et al. Molecular pathogenesis of anti-NMDAR encephalitis. Biomed Res Int. 2015;2015:643409.
9. D'Andrea M. Add Alzheimer's disease to the list of autoimmune diseases. Medical Hypotheses. 2005;64(3):458-63.
10. Geschwind MD, Tan KM, Lennon VA, et al. Voltage-gated potassium channel autoimmunity mimicking Creutzfeldt-Jakob disease. Arch Neurol. 2008;65:1341-6.
11. Gonzales-Portillo F, McIntyre JA, Wagenknecht DR, et al. Spectrum of antiphospholipid antibodies (aPL) in patients with cerebrovascular disease. J Stroke Cerebrovasc Dis. 2001;10:222-6.
12. Hanly JG, Hong C, Smith S, et al. A prospective analysis of cognitive function and anticardiolipin antibodies in systemic lupus erythematosus. Arthritis Rheum. 1999;42:728-34.
13. Hara M, Ariño H, Petit-Pedrol M, et al. DPPX antibody–associated encephalitis Main syndrome and antibody effects. Neurology. 2017;88:1340-8.
14. Höftberger R, Titulaer MJ, Sabater L, et al. Encephalitis and GABAB receptor antibodies novel findings in a new case series of 20 patients. Neurology. 2013;81:1500-6.
15. Höftberger R, van Sonderen A, Leypoldt F, et al. Encephalitis and AMPA receptor antibodies novel findings in a case series of 22 patients. Neurology. 2015;84:2403-12.
16. Joubert B, Kerschen P, Zekeridou A, et al. Clinical spectrum of encephalitis associated with antibodies against the α-amino-3-hydroxy-5-methyl-4-isoxazolepropionic acid receptor: Case series and review of the literature. JAMA Neurol. 2015;72(10):1163-9.
17. Kemp M, Kimber J, Zhang L. Anti-voltage gated potassium channel (VGKC) antibody positive encephalopathy. J Neurol Neurosurg Psychiatry. 2015;86:e4..
18. Lai M, Hughes EG, Peng X, et al. AMPA receptor antibodies in limbic encephalitis alter synaptic receptor location. Ann Neurol. 2009;65(4):424-34.
19. Lancaster E, Dalmau J. Neuronal autoantigens—pathogenesis, associated disorders and antibody testing. Nat Rev Neurol. 2012;8(7):380-90.
20. Lehrer S, Rheinstein P. Is Alzheimer's disease autoimmune inflammation of the brain that can be treated with nasal nonsteroidal anti-inflammatory drugs? Am J Alzheimers Dis Other Demen. 2014;30(3):225-7.
21. Liu CY, Zhu J, Zheng XY, et al. Anti-N-methyl-D-aspartate receptor encephalitis: A severe, potentially reversible autoimmune encephalitis Mediators Inflamm. 2017;2017:6361479.
22. Luyendijk J, Steens SC, Ouwendijk WJ, et al. Neuropsychiatric systemic lupus erythematosus: Lessons learned from magnetic resonance imaging. Arthritis Rheum. 2011;63:722-32.
23. Manto MU, Laute MA, Aguera M, et al. Effects of anti–glutamic acid decarboxylase antibodies associated with neurological diseases. Ann Neurol. 2007;61(6):544-51.
24. Martinez-Martinez P, Molenaar PC, Losen M, et al. Glycine receptor antibodies in PERM: A new channelopathy. Brain. 2014;137:2115-6.
25. McGeer PL, Schulzer M, McGeer EG. Arthritis and anti-inflammatory agents as possible protective factors for Alzheimer's disease: A review of 17 epidemiologic studies. Neurology. 1996;47:425-32.

26. McKeon A, Lennon VA, Lachance DH, et al. Ganglionic acetylcholine receptor autoantibody: Oncological, neurological, and serological accompaniments. Arch Neurol. 2009;66:735-41.
27. McKeon A. Autoimmune encephalopathies and dementias. Continuum (Minneap Minn). 2016;22(2 Dementia):538-58.
28. Miller BL, Boeve BF (Eds). The Behavioral Neurology of Dementia. Cambridge, UK: Cambridge University Press; 2016.
29. Miller Z, Rankin K, Graff-Radford N, et al. TDP-43 frontotemporal lobar degeneration and autoimmune disease. J Neurol Neurosurg Psychiatry. 2013;84(9):956-62.
30. Misawa T, Mizusawa H. Anti-VGKC antibody-associated limbic encephalitis/Morvan syndrome. Brain Nerve. 2010;62:339-45.
31. Muscal E, Traipe E, de Guzman MM, et al. Cerebral and cerebellar volume loss in children and adolescents with systemic lupus erythematosus: A review of clinically acquired brain magnetic resonance imaging. J Rheumatol. 2010;37:1768-75.
32. Piepgras J, Höltje M, Michel K, et al. Anti-DPPX encephalitis pathogenic effects of antibodies on gut and brain neurons. Neurology. 2015;85:890-7.
33. Rosenbloom MH, Smith S, Akdal G, et al. Immunologically mediated dementias. Current Neurol Neurosci Rep. 2009;9:359-67.
34. Schmitt SE, Pargeon K, Frechette ES, et al. Extreme delta brush: A unique EEG pattern in adults with anti-NMDA receptor encephalitis. Neurology. 2012;79(11):1094-100.
35. Tobin WO, Pittock SJ. Autoimmune neurology of the central nervous system. Continuum (Minneap Minn). 2017;23:627-53.
36. Wolkowitz OM, Lupien SJ, Bigler ED. The steroid dementia syndrome: A possible model of human glucocorticoid neurotoxicity. Neurocase. 2007;13:189-200.
37. Wotton C, Goldacre M. Associations between specific autoimmune diseases and subsequent dementia: retrospective record-linkage cohort study, UK. J Epidemiol Community Health. 2017;71(6):576-83.
38. Wyss-Coray T, Rogers J. Inflammation in Alzheimer disease-a brief review of the basic science and clinical literature. Cold Spring Harb Perspect Med. 2012;2(1):a006346.

CHAPTER 5

Autoimmune Demyelinating Disorders

Mugundhan Krishnan, Lakshmi Narasimhan Ranganathan, Chandramouleeswaran V, Mariappan V, Balasubramanian Samivel, Ganesh Veeraraghavan

INTRODUCTION

Autoimmune demyelination of central nervous system (CNS) is characterized by immune mediated damage to various cells, which include the myelin covering nerve cells in brain, spinal cord, and peripheral nerves as a result of loss of anergy to the self-antigenicity. In this chapter, the three autoimmune demyelinating diseases are dealt in detail—multiple sclerosis (MS), neuromyelitis optica (NMO), and acute disseminated encephalomyelitis (ADEM).

MULTILPLE SCLEROSIS

Multiple sclerosis is an autoimmune inflammatory demyelinating disease of CNS.

Pathogenesis

The major pathogenesis involves chronic inflammation with perivenular accumulation of T lymphocytes and macrophages resulting in disruption of blood–brain barrier followed by demyelination, secondary axonal degeneration, and plaque formation. Major histocompatibility complex (MHC) class I and class II alleles are involved in the T-cell activation and regulation. Increased expression of interleukin (IL)-23, myelin-reactive T-cells in plaques and immunoglobulin (Ig) G oligoclonal bands in cerebrospinal fluid (CSF) are associated with active MS. The primary event preceding inflammation is oligodendrocyte apoptosis which is triggered by viral infection or glutamate excitotoxicity.

Epidemiology and Risk Factors

Male to female ratio is 2.5:1, with incidence and prevalence varying geographically. The mean age of onset is around 27–32 years with relapsing-remitting multiple sclerosis (RRMS) has earlier onset than primary progressive multiple sclerosis (PPMS). More than 100 polymorphisms are associated with MS, the strongest association is with human leukocyte antigen (HLA)-DRB1*15 and *16 and protective effect is noted with HLA-DRB1*04, *07 and *09. Polymorphisms in B-cell activating factor has a strong correlation with MS. Lifetime risk of MS is increased by 6-fold among first-degree relatives. Environmental factors influencing MS includes viral infections with Epstein-Barr virus (EBV), geographical location in temperate countries, vitamin D deficiency, and babies born in April and May.

Clinical Features

There are no specific clinical features unique to MS.
- Bowel and bladder dysfunction (50–70%): Detrusor overactivity, detrusor sphincter dyssynergia, and fecal incontinence
- Cognitive impairment (5%): Depression is more common in MS with increased risk of suicide
- Epilepsy (2%)
- Eye movement disorders (35–40%): Internuclear ophthalmoplegia, one-and-a-half syndrome, pendular and periodic alternating nystagmus, disorders of smooth pursuit system
- Fatigue (85%)
- Heat sensitivity (60–80%)
- Motor symptoms (35%)
- Spasticity (30%)
- Pain (65%)
- Sensory symptoms (37%): Numbness and paresthesia
- Sexual dysfunction (50%)
- Sleep disorders (50–60%): Restless leg syndrome, obstructive sleep apnea syndrome
- Vertigo (30–50%)
- Optic neuritis (ON) (90%)
- Ancillary symptoms: Trigeminal neuralgia, Lhermitte's sign.

Disease Course

1. Relapsing-remitting MS (85%): Characterized by relapses with full recovery or with residual sequelae. Relapsing-remitting multiple sclerosis will subsequently enter into secondary-progressive multiple sclerosis (SPMS) (Fig. 1)
2. Secondary-progressive MS: Steady decline in function not associated with acute attacks. Transition from RRMS to SPMS is around 2% per year (Fig. 2)
3. Primary-progressive MS (10%): Steady decline in function from disease onset without acute attacks (Fig. 3)
4. Progressive/relapsing MS (5%): Steady decline in function from disease onset with occasional attacks superimposed on progressive course (Fig. 4).

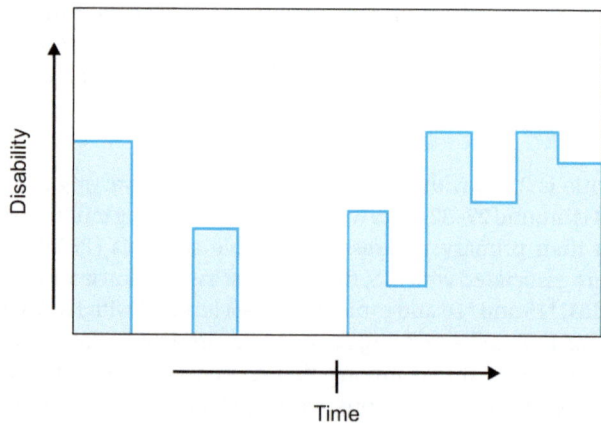

FIG. 1: Relapsing-remitting multiple sclerosis.

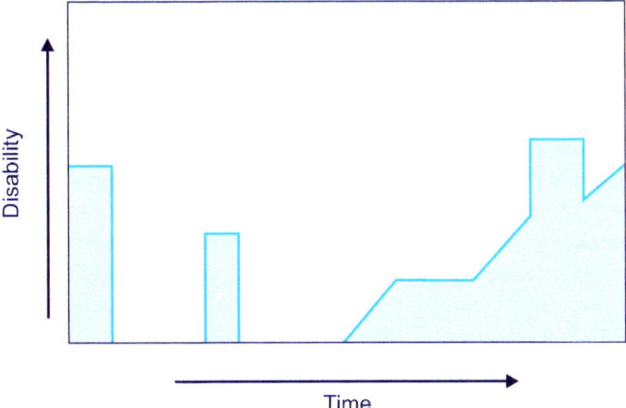
FIG. 2: Secondary-progressive multiple sclerosis.

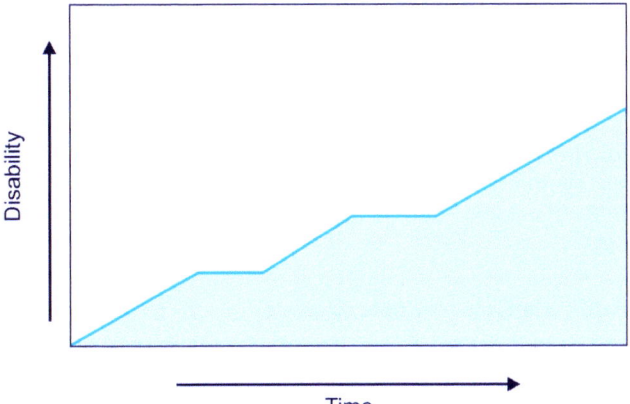
FIG. 3: Primary-progressive multiple sclerosis.

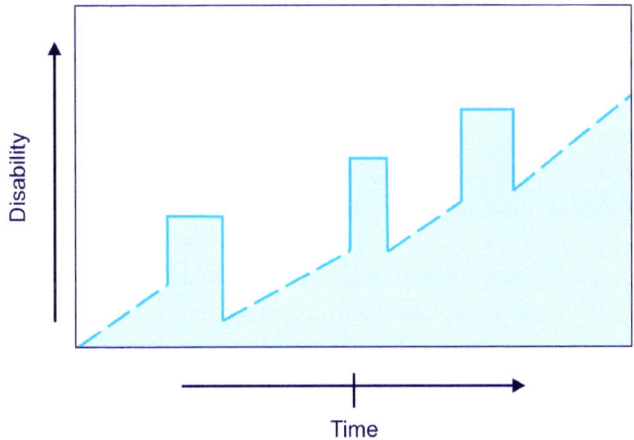
FIG. 4: Progressive/relapsing multiple sclerosis.

Diagnosis

There is no definite test for diagnosis for MS.

Imaging

Magnetic resonance imaging (MRI) remains the test of choice to support clinical diagnosis and better predictor of progression to definite MS than CSF. Plaques in MRI suggesting of MS are found in periventicular region, corpus callosum, centrum semiovale and deeper white matter. Breakdown of blood-brain barrier, resulting in vascular permeability, is detected by leakage of gadolinium-diethylenetriamine penta-acetic acid into the brain parenchyma. Lesions are oriented perpendicular to the ventricles (Dawson's finger). Gadolinium enhancing lesions in T1W MRI often correspond to areas of high signal on T2W MRI and low signal on unenhanced T1W images. Black holes in T1W are considered as markers of severe demyelination.

Proton magnetic resonance spectroscopy measures metabolic components such as N-acetyl aspartate and creatine ratio, which serves as a marker for neuronal loss. Diffusion tensor imaging measures fractional anisotropy which differentiates edema from demyelination. Diagnostic criteria for MS was first developed by Poser in 1980, later it was supplanted by McDonald criteria developed in 2001, modified in 2005 and revised again in 2010 (Table 1).

Cerebrospinal Fluid Analysis

Cerebrospinal fluid in MS shows mononuclear pleocytosis with normal protein. Increased intrathecal protein synthesis measured by CSF IgG index is found in 90% of definite MS. Cerebrospinal fluid oligoclonal band measured by agarose gel electrophoresis is found in 95% of definite MS.

TABLE 1: McDonald's criteria for multiple sclerosis

Clinical features	Additional requirements
Attacks >2 OR Lesions >2 clinically OR one lesion with history of of prior attack	NONE
Attacks >2; one lesion clinically	Dissemination in space: One or more T2 lesions in 2/4 MS typical regions OR Awaiting further attack in different CNS site
One attack; lesions >2 clinically	Dissemination in time: Asymptomatic gadolinium enhancing and nonenhancing lesions simultaneously at any time OR new T2 lesion on follow-up MRI or awaiting a second attack
PPMS	One year of disease progression plus 2/3 of the following: Positive CSF OCB/elevated IgG index, Dissemination in space in brain with one or more T2 lesion, dissemination in space in spinal cord with two or more T2 lesions

OCB, oligoclonal band; CSF, cerebrospinal fluid; CNS, central nervous system; MS, multiple sclerosis; MRI, magnetic resonance imaging; PPMS, primary progressive multiple sclerosis; IgG, immunoglobulin G.

TABLE 2: Subclinical abnormalities in central nervous system function

Test	Abnormalities (%)
Visual evoked potential	50–90
Brainstem evoked response audiometry	20–55
Somatosensory evoked potential	50

Evoked Potential
Detects subclinical abnormalities in CNS function (Table 2).

Treatment
Therapy for MS is divided into four categories.

Acute Attacks
Intravenous pulse methylprednisolone 500–1000 mg for 3–5 days followed by oral prednisolone 40–60 mg tapered over a period of 14 days. Plasmapheresis (5–6 exchanges, dose of 40–60 mL/kg) may be used in patients with fulminant demyelination not responsive to steroids.

Disease Modifying Drugs
They reduce the relapse rate and delay the progression of brain lesions on MRI.
None of the drug completely cures the disease. Responses to therapy are assessed with expanded disability status scale every 3 months and MRI brain every 12 months (Flowchart 1).

Injectable Therapy
- Interferons: First disease modifying therapy (DMT) approved for MS. Acts by downregulation of MHC molecules on antigen-presenting cell (APC), reducing inflammatory cytokines, and limiting the trafficking of lymphocytes into CNS
    - Interferon beta-1a, (intramuscular) 30 µg once a week
    - Interferon beta-1a, (subcutaneous) 44 µg thrice weekly
    - Interferon beta-1b, (subcutaneous) 250 µg every other day
    - Pegylated interferon B-1a, (subcutaneous) 125 mg once every 2 weeks.
- Glatiramer acetate: It is a synthetic polypeptide, antigenically similar to myelin basic protein. Acts by displacing the bound myelin basic protein by binding to MHC molecules and expression of anti-inflammatory cytokines. Given by subcutaneous injection at 20 mg or 40 mg thrice weekly
- Daclizumab: Humanized monoclonal antibody binds to alpha chain of subcutaneous receptor. Highly effective against reducing relapse rate in RRMS, approved by Food and Drug Administration in 2016. Given by subcutaneous injection, 150 mg once a month.

Infusion Therapies
- Natalizumab: Humanized monoclonal antibody acts against alpha 4 subunit of $\alpha4\beta1$ integrin, on the surface of lymphocytes. Highly effective in reducing attack rate and disease severity. The risk of progressive multifocal leukoencephalopathy with natalizumab is 4.1/1000 per year. Anti-John Cunningham virus antibodies are advised

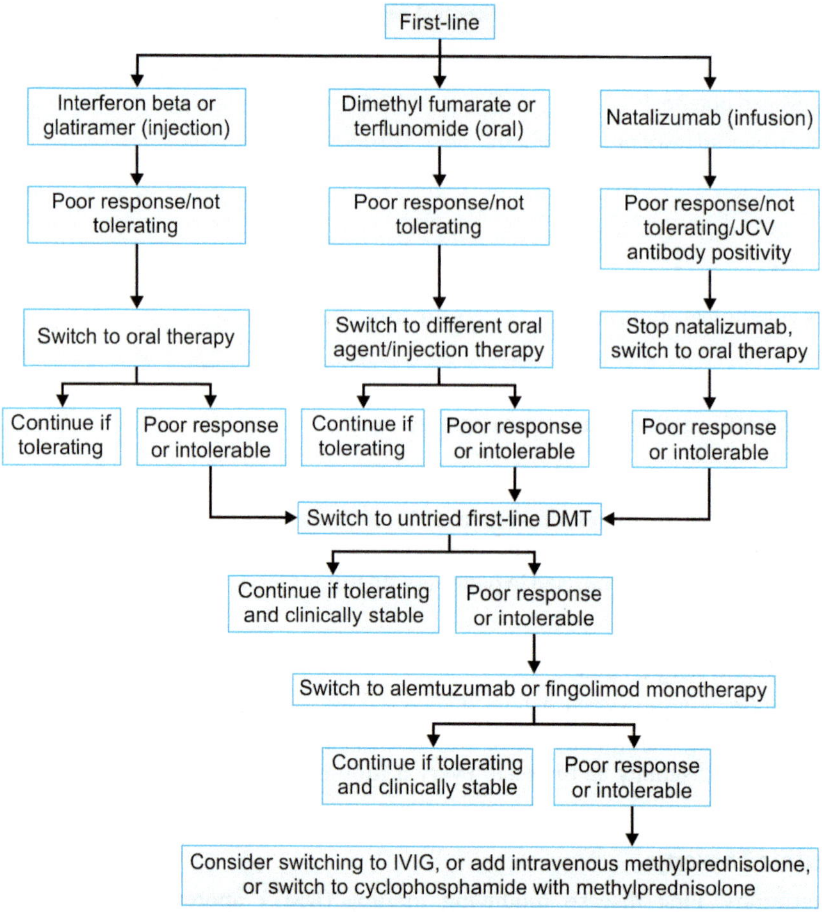

Immune-mediated Neurological Disorders

FLOWCHART 1: Disease modifying drugs for refractory relapsing-remitting multiple sclerosis.

DMT, disease modifying therapy; IVIG, intravenous immunoglobulin; JCV, John Cunningham virus.

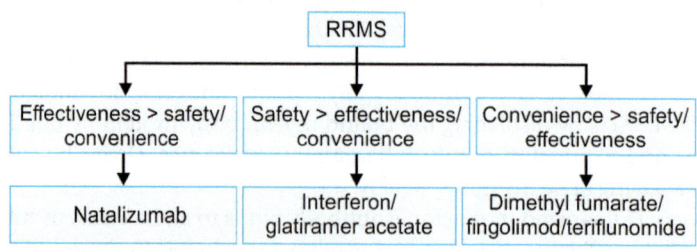

RRMS, relapsing-remitting multiple sclerosis.

FLOWCHART 2: Initial drugs for RRMS.

one year after therapy with natalizumab. Administered at a dose of 300 mg intravenous infusion every 4 weeks (Flowchart 2)
- Alemtuzumab: Humanized monoclonal antibody causing depletion of CD52 expression on T-cells, B-cells, natural killer cells, and monocytes. More effective than

interferon in reducing the relapse rate. Given by intravenous infusion at 12 mg daily for 5 days (totally 60 mg) followed by 12 mg daily for 3 days (totally 36 mg) after 12 months
- Ocrelizumab: Recombinant human monoclonal antibody directed against anti-CD20, causing depletion of B-cells by antibody dependent cell mediated cytotoxicity and complement dependent cytotoxicity. First drug effective against PPMS, reduces gadolinium enhancing brain lesions by 90%. Initial dose of ocrelizumab is given as 300 mg intravenous infusion, followed 2 weeks later by second 300 mg intravenous infusion and further doses are given as 600 mg intravenous infusion every 6 months
- Mitoxantrone: Anti-cancer drug acts by producing DNA strand breaks, decreasing RNA synthesis and inhibiting topoisomerase II. Approved for use in both RRMS and SPMS. Dosing schedules are 12 mg/m$_2$ every 3 months, with maximum duration of therapy for 2-3 years.

Oral Therapies

- Dimethyl fumarate: Neuroprotective, antioxidant, and immunomodulatory drug acts by modulation of expression of proinflammatory and anti-inflammatory cytokines. Starting dose is 120 mg twice daily for 7 days followed by 240 mg twice daily
- Teriflunomide: Inhibits pyrimidine biosynthesis and prevents the interaction of T-cells with APC. Given at a dose of 7-14 mg once daily for 2 years. Highly teratogenic and pregnancy should be avoided until serum concentration is less than 0.02 mg/L
- Fingolimod: Sphingosine-1-phosphate inhibitor and prevents the migration of lymphocytes from secondary lymphoid organs. Effective in RRMS given at a dose of 0.5 mg daily.

Other Therapies

- Azathioprine (AZA)
- Rituximab
- Cyclophosphamide
- Cladribine
- Dalfampridine
- Intravenous immunoglobulin
- Laquinimod
- Autologous stem cell transplantation.

Pregnancy and Multiple Sclerosis

The overall disease course is unaffected, as fewer attacks are experienced during gestation, with more attacks expected in the first 3 months postpartum. Disease modifying therapy is usually discontinued during pregnancy. Acute attacks are treated with intravenous methylprednisolone.

NEUROMYELITIS OPTICA

Neuromyelitis optica is an autoimmune inflammatory disorder of CNS that preferentially affects the optic nerves and spinal cord. It was formerly known as Devic's disease, a severe variant of MS. It has distinctive and specific clinical, radiological and pathological features. Neuromyelitis optica and its limited forms are known as NMO spectrum disorders (NMOSD). Most NMOSD are associated with antibodies to aquaporin-4 channel

(AQP-4 IgG). In fewer percentages of AQP-4 seronegative cases, it is associated with myelin oligodendrocytic glycoprotein antibody (MOG Ab).

Epidemiology

Neuromyelitis optica occurs in all major ethnic groups, with prevalence of 0.5 and 10 per 1,00,000. It has a strong female predilection as in other autoimmune disorders with female to male ratios ranging from 2:1 to 10:1. The median age of onset is 39 years, but the disease also occurs in children and elderly. Its prevalence is high in Asia and West Indies and low in North America and Australia.

Neuromyelitis optica is a sporadic disease, but familial cases can also occur (3% of patients). Human leukocyte antigens associated with high risk includes DRB1*0301 in white people and DP B1*0501 in Asians.

Clinical Presentation

The classic clinical manifestation of NMO is recurrent acute attacks of unilateral or bilateral ON and/or transverse myelitis (TM) with incomplete recovery between attacks. Relapsing course is seen in 90% of patients and remaining 10% have monophasic course. Around 60% of the patients experience a relapse within 1 year and 90% within 3 years after the first attack. Particularly, patients who are NMO-AQP-4 seropositive with recurrent ON or the first episode of longitudinally extensive transverse myelitis (LETM) are at high risk of relapse. Various limited forms have been recently included which are described below.

Optic Neuritis

It typically presents with reduced visual acuity and eye pain aggravated by eye movements. Patients of simultaneous bilateral ON or severe ON with poor recovery despite treatment and noncentral scotoma deficits such as altitudinal field defects should raise suspicion. The lesions are typically longer involving more than half the length of optic nerve and involve the posterior aspect of the nerve or the chiasm.

Magnetic resonance imaging may show increased signal on fat suppressed T2-weighted sequences or T1 gadolinium enhancement in the optic nerve or optic chiasm.

Transverse Myelitis

Transverse myelitis is characterized by severe spinal cord dysfunction which often results in complete spinal cord syndrome (c.f. with MS) with paraparesis or quadriparesis, bladder dysfunction, and sensory loss caudal to the level of the cord lesion. Pain is particularly prominent. Recovery may be poor despite treatment.

Magnetic resonance imaging shows LETM, lesions extending over three or more spinal cord segments, involving the cervical or thoracic cord. Cervical lesions extending into the medulla have high predictive value for NMOSD. Lesions preferentially involve the central gray matter which usually show enhancement with gadolinium (c.f. with MS) (Fig. 5).

Acute Brainstem Syndrome

This occurs frequently (34%). The common symptoms are vomiting (33%), hiccups (22%), oculomotor dysfunction (20%), and pruritus (12%). Less common symptoms include hearing loss, facial palsy, vertigo, vestibular ataxia, and trigeminal neuralgia. Lesions are typically periependymal.

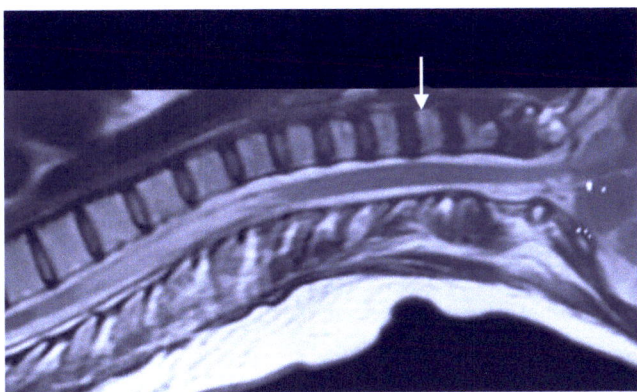

FIG. 5: T2-magnetic resonance imaging of neuromyelitis optica spectrum disorder patient showing central hyperintensity extending from C1 to D4.

Area Postrema Syndrome

It is characterized by intractable hiccups and/or nausea and vomiting (43%). It may be the presenting manifestation in up to 10% of the cases. Magnetic resonance imaging shows lesions involving dorsal medulla (especially area postrema). It shows good response to steroids.

Acute Diencephalic Syndrome

It may manifest with various endocrinopathies like syndrome of inappropriate antidiuretic hormone secretion, narcolepsy, hypo or hyperthermia, anorexia or obesity, hyperprolactinemia. Magnetic resonance imaging shows lesions in hypothalamus and areas adjacent to basilar cistern or the third ventricle.

Symptomatic Cerebral Syndrome

It may present in the form of encephalopathy (large hemispheric lesions), posterior reversible encephalopathy syndrome or focal neurological deficits.

Diagnostic Evaluation

The initial diagnostic evaluation should include serologic testing for AQP-4-IgG, CSF analysis and neuroimaging of the brain and spine with MRI.

Serum Aquaporin 4–Immunoglobulin G Testing

It is a specific NMO biomarker and plays an essential role in the disease pathogenesis. Serum AQP-4 antibodies have 73% sensitivity and 91% specificity for clinically defined NMO. Sensitivity depends on analytical methods used for the detection of AQP-4-IgG and is highest for cell-based assays. Around 10–25% of NMO patients are seronegative for AQP-4-IgG. Antibodies against MOG are found in fraction of AQP-4 seronegative patients. In contrast with AQP-4 positive patients, MOG positive patients have higher frequency of simultaneous ON, milder TM of cervical or lumbosacral cord, and better prognosis.

Cerebrospinal Fluid Examination

Cerebrospinal fluid studies should include cell count, cytology, protein, albumin CSF–serum ratio, immunoglobulin (IgG, IgA, IgM) CSF–serum ratios, and oligoclonal bands. It is helpful in distinguishing NMOSD from MS. Significant pleocytosis (>50 cells/mm^3) with a high proportion of neutrophils and high protein level (100–500 mg/dL) is common in NMO, unlike in MS. Oligoclonal IgG bands are present in 85–90% of patients with MS, but are uncommon in patients with NMO (15–30%). The albumin quotient may be elevated, particularly during a relapse, indicating blood–brain barrier disruption. Glial fibrillary acidic protein is significantly elevated which reflects prominent astrocyte damage unique of NMOSD. Cerebrospinal fluid IL-6 is elevated which is not observed in MS.

Neuroimaging

Patients should undergo MRI with and without gadolinium enhancement of the brain and spine, as well as optic nerve MRI in cases suspicious of ON. Imaging features associated with the most common clinical syndromes are described in the "Clinical Presentation" section. Brain MRI may reveal nonspecific deep white matter lesions which are typically extensive with irregular and indistinct borders and are clinically silent. Acute brain lesions show different contrast enhancement patterns like "cloudlike", "pencil thin" and rarely meningeal enhancement.

Diagnostic Criteria

The International Panel for Neuromyelitis Optica Diagnosis (IPND) revised the diagnostic criteria and published it in 2015. The new criteria unifies the concepts of NMO and NMOSD and stratifies it further into seropositive and seronegative types. Diagnosis is based on the presence of "six core clinical characteristics", AQP-4 antibody status, and MRI imaging features. More stringent clinical criteria with additional neuroimaging features are required for seronegative NMO diagnosis. These criteria are highlighted in Box 1.

According to IPND, NMOSD diagnosis can be made only when the patient has experienced at least one clinical attack. Asymptomatic seropositivity for AQP-4-IgG or asymptomatic MRI lesions characteristic for NMOSD are insufficient for the diagnosis.

Treatment

Treatment recommendations are based upon data from observational studies and by the consensus from clinical experience of experts.

Acute Attacks

Neuromyelitis optica spectrum disorder patients with acute attacks, both initial and recurrent should be treated as soon as possible. Initial treatment with high-dose intravenous methylprednisolone (1 g daily for 3–5 consecutive days) is usually given. Plasma exchange is indicated in patients with severe symptoms unresponsive to steroids and usually done on alternative days up to a total of seven exchanges.

Maintenance Therapy

There is no well-established or optimal therapy for the maintenance of remission and prevention of relapse. Observational studies show improved outcomes with several immunosuppressive agents, including rituximab, mycophenolate mofetil, AZA, and

Box 1: Diagnostic criteria for neuromyelitis optica spectrum disorders

Core clinical characteristics
- Optic neuritis
- Acute myelitis
- Area postrema syndrome (episodes of otherwise unexplained hiccups or nausea and vomiting)
- Acute braintem syndrome
- Symptomatic narcolepsy or acute diencephalic clinical syndrome with NMOSD-typical diencephalic MRI lesions
- Symptomatic cerebral syndrome with NMOSD-typical brain lesions

Diagnostic criteria for NMOSD with aquaporin 4-immunoglobuin G (AQP-4-IgG)
- At least 1 core clinical characteristic
- Positive test for AQP-4-IgG using best available detection method
- Exclusion of alternative diagnoses

Diagnostic criteria for NMOSD without AQP-4-IgG or antibody status unknown
- At least 2 core clinical characteristics meeting all of the following characteristics:
  - At least 1 core clinical characteristic must be optic neuritis, acute myelitis with LETM, or area postrema syndrome
  - Dissemination in space (two or more different core clinical characteristics)
  - Fulfillment of additional MRI requirements
    - Acute optic neuritis: Brain MRI shows normal findings or nonspecific white matter lesions; OR optic nerve MRI demonstrates T2-hyperintense lesion or T1-weighted gadolinium enhancing lesion extending over at least half the optic nerve length or involving optic chiasm
    - Acute myelitis: Spine MRI lesion extending over at least three contiguous segments (LETM)
    - Area postrema syndrome: Associated dorsal medulla lesions
    - Acute brainstem syndrome: Associated periependymal brainstem lesions
- Negative test for AQP-4-IgG, or testing unavailable
- Exclusion of alternative diagnoses

NMOSDs, neuromyelitis optica spectrum disorders; LETM, longitudinally extensive transverse myelitis; MRI, magnetic resonance imaging; IgM, immunoglobulin M.

mitoxantrone. Initial and maintenance treatment of seronegative disease is similar to the seropositive disease.

ACUTE DISSEMINATED ENCEPHALOMYELITIS

Acute disseminated encephalomyelitis is an autoimmune demyelinating disease of CNS which is characterized by rapid onset polyfocal neurological symptoms including encephalopathy. In 2013, the International Pediatric Multiple Sclerosis Study Group updated new criteria for diagnosis of ADEM which is given below. Though, ADEM is a monophasic illness, in subset of patients, it is followed by another relapse or evolved into multiple sclerosis and NMO.

Diagnostic Criteria (Table 3)
Monophasic ADEM
- Single polyfocal CNS event with presumed inflammatory demyelinating cause
- Encephalopathy, which is unexplained by fever, postictal symptoms or systemic illness
- Magnetic resonance imaging brain abnormalities consistent with demyelination during the acute phase
- There is no new MRI findings or clinical symptoms after the clinical onset of 3 months or more.

Pathogenesis
Though its pathogenesis is incompletely understood, the proposed mechanism is triggering of immune system by an environmental stimuli (infections, vaccination) in genetically susceptible individuals. Myelin basic protein, myelin oligodendrocyte protein and proteolipid protein of myelinated axons in CNS share its antigenic property with infectious agent (molecular mimicry).

Pathology
The typical pathology findings in ADEM is perivenular sleeves of demyelination and inflammation. Acute disseminated encephalomyelitis lesions are of same histologic age and larger lesions are formed by coalescence of numerous perivenular demyelinating lesions. Hemorrhagic demyelination of CNS is considered to be hyperacute form of ADEM. These hyperacute variants include acute hemorrhagic leukoencephalitis, acute hemorrhagic encephalomyelitis and acute necrotizing hemorrhagic leukoencephalitis (Weston-Hurst syndrome).

Epidemiology
Acute disseminated encephalomyelitis can occur at any age but predominantly affects children of 5–8 years with slight male preponderance. It is an uncommon illness and is often precipitated by infection or vaccination. The estimated incidence in Canada is 0.2/1,00,000 and in California and Japan is 0.4/100,000 per year. Nonspecific upper

TABLE 3: Acute disseminated encephalomyelitis relapse classification

Diagnosis	Clinical criteria
MDEM	ADEM followed at >3 months by second ADEM episode, but no further ADEM or non-ADEM demyelinating events
ADEM-MS	ADEM followed at >3 months by non-ADEM demyelinating relapse and new MRI lesions meeting criteria for dissemination in space
ADEM-NMOSD	ADEM followed at >3 months by events including optic neuritis, longitudinally extensive transverse myelitis, or area postrema syndrome meeting MRI requirements according to revised NMOSD criteria
ADEM-ON	ADEM, MDEM, or multiple ADEM attacks followed by optic neuritis

ON, optic neuritis; MDEM, multiphasic disseminated encephalomyelitis; NMOSD, neuromyelitis optica spectrum disorder; MS, multiple sclerosis; ADEM, Acute disseminated encephalomyelitis, MRI, magnetic resonance imaging.

respiratory tract infections present in 50–70% of children in the 4 weeks prior to onset of neurological symptoms. Organisms that have been implicated in postinfectious ADEM include EBV, measles, herpes simplex virus, varicella zoster virus, cytomegalovirus, human immunodeficiency virus, hepatitis A and *Mycoplasma pneumoniae*. Less than 5% of cases are related to vaccine. Postvaccinial ADEM is seen in association with rabies, pertussis, rubella, measles, chicken pox and diphtheria vaccine. Currently, the incidence of postvaccinial ADEM is reduced and it is 1 to 2 per 1 million vaccination.

Clinical Features

The course of illness is rapid with multifocal neurological deficit occuring in 2–5 days. Prodromal symptoms including fever, malaise, irritability, somnolence, headache and vomiting can occur sometimes. Neurological manifestations include acute onset encephalopathy, seizures, pyramidal signs, ataxia, cranial nerve palsies, ON, speech impairment, hemiparesis, spinal cord syndrome and respiratory failure. This acute illness usually lasts for 2–4 weeks and many develop new neurological symptoms and signs. After an acute phase, most of the children will have complete recovery spontaneously and some may have residual neurological deficit mostly affecting cognition. The mortality rate during acute phase is reported to be 1–3%. Hemorrhagic variants are more severe than typical ADEM and recovery of neurology function is worse.

Diagnosis

There is no specific test to diagnose ADEM and diagnosis is based on clinical, MRI and other investigations to exclude other differential diagnoses. Cerebrospinal fluid analysis including cell count, sugar, protein, lactate, oligoclonal bands, IgG index, culture and viral markers need to be done to differentiate demyelination from treatable CNS infections. Cerebrospinal fluid findings in ADEM show evidence of inflammation with mild pleocytosis (<50 cells) and/or mild increased protein concentration (<100 mg). Oligoclonal bands can present occasionally in CSF but more commonly associated with multiple sclerosis. Magnetic resonance imaging of brain typically demonstrate multiple hyperintense lesions involving bilateral subcortical, central white matter, cortical gray-white matter junction, thalami, basal ganglia, cerebellum and brain stem in T2-weighted and FLAIR images. Bilateral diffuse lesions, poorly defined lesions, large globular lesions, periventricular sparing, absence of Dawson fingers are some of the differentiating features of ADEM from MS. Complete or partial resolution is seen in follow-up MRI in ADEM. Hemorrhagic variants show red blood cells in CSF and hemorrhage in spin-echo MRI sequence along with ADEM findings.

Treatment

High dose corticosteroid is the mainstay of treatment. Intravenous methylprednisolone (10–30 mg/kg per day, maximum 1,000 mg daily) or dexamethasone (1 mg/kg per day) for 5 days followed by oral steroid tapered over 4–6 weeks. Intravenous Ig and plasma exchange act as rescue therapy for those who fail to respond to steroid.

CONCLUSION

Autoimmune demyelinating diseases of brain and spinal cord are chronic, require lifelong care and frequent monitoring. Support groups like Multiple Sclerosis Foundation Society are all helpful in informing the patients about the nature of the disease and how to cope with their diseases smoothly.

TAKE HOME MESSAGES

- The number of available DMT has increased greatly over the past decade and each patient to be assessed effectively for receiving appropriate therapy
- Symptomatic therapy for MS is an important aspect of management
- The new NMOSD diagnostic criteria (seropositive and seronegative NMOSD) paves a new era in clinical practice which allows an easier and homogenous diagnosis
- NMOSD is distinct from MS, has poor prognosis and leads to permanent neurological disability. Hence, an early diagnosis and effective treatment is essential.
- Though ADEM is previously considered as monophasic, it can evolve in to multiphasic ADEM, MS or NMO in small set of patients
- Early recognition and treatment of ADEM with steroids carry a good prognosis.

SUGGESTED READINGS

1. Brownlee WJ, Hardy TA, Fazekas F, et al. Diagnosis of multiple sclerosis: Progress and challenges. Lancet. 2017;389:1336.
2. Cabre P, Olindo S, Marignier R, et al. Efficacy of mitoxantrone in neuromyelitis optica spectrum: Clinical and neuroradiological study. J Neurol Neurosurg Psychiatry. 2013;84:511.
3. Capra R, Cordioli C, Rasia S, et al. Assessing long term prognosis improvement as a consequence of treatment in MS. Mult Scler. 2017;23(13):1757-61.
4. Dasgupta R, Fowler CJ. Bladder, bowel and sexual dysfunction in MS: Management strategies. Drugs Rev. 2003;63:153.
5. Davis LE, Booss J. Acute disseminated encephalomyelitis in children: A changing picture. Pediatr Infect Dis J. 2003;22:829.
6. Dendrou CA, Fugger L, Friese MA. Immunopathology of MS. Nat Rev Immunol. 2015;15:545.
7. Filippi M, Rocca MA. MR imaging of multiple sclerosis. Radiology. 2011;259:659.
8. Hinson SR, McKeon A, Lennon VA. Neurological autoimmunity targeting aquaporin-4. Neuroscience. 2010;168:1009.
9. Hynson JL, Kornberg AJ, Coleman LT, et al. Clinical and neuroradiologic features of acute disseminated encephalomyelitis in children. Neurology. 2001;56:1308.
10. Krupp LB, Tardieu M, Amato MP, et al. International Pediatric Multiple Sclerosis Study Group criteria for pediatric multiple sclerosis and immune-mediated central nervous system demyelinating disorders: Revisions to the 2007 definitions. Mult Scler. 2013;19:1261.
11. Papadopoulos MC, Verkman AS. Aquaporin 4 and neuromyelitis optica. Lancet Neurol. 2012;11:535.
12. Sellner J, Boggild M, Clanet M, et al. EFNS guidelines on diagnosis and management of neuromyelitis optica. Eur J Neurol. 2010;17:1019.
13. Stonehouse M, Gupte G, Wassmer E, et al. Acute disseminated encephalomyelitis: Recognition in the hands of general paediatricians. Arch Dis Child. 2003;88:122.
14. Wingerchuk DM, Cabrera-Gómez JA, Kurtzke JF, et al. An epidemiological study of neuromyelitis optica in Cuba. J Neurol. 2009;256:35.

CHAPTER 6

Autoimmune Epilepsies

Afshan Jabeen Shaik, Manjeera Sri Padma K

INTRODUCTION

The etiology of epilepsies still remains elusive in majority of epilepsies, many of which are resistant to treatment with antiepileptic drugs (AEDs). The discovery of autoantibodies and the response to immunotherapy in patients with seizure disorder lead to the description of autoimmune epilepsies. In this chapter, the authors review the current understanding of autoimmune epilepsies.

HISTORICAL ASPECTS

The concept of antibody-associated central nervous system (CNS) disorders appeared for the first time in 1960. The first description of autoimmune epilepsies was in 1960s in association with Hashimoto's thyroiditis. Later in 1980s, there was discovery of anti-GAD antibodies and antibodies against onconeural antigens, which were typically of paraneoplastic etiology. The discovery of antibodies against surface antigens [N-methyl-D-aspartate (NMDA) receptor, voltage-gated potassium channel (VGKC)] was a breakthrough in neurology, as these epilepsies and encephalitis tend to have good response to immunotherapy.

Approximately, three-quarters of CNS disorders with antibodies to surface antigens present with epileptic seizures. Clinical features in antibody-associated "autoimmune epilepsies" may not always be absolutely typical for the described clinical syndromes, but still be responsive to immunological therapies.

The antibodies can cause both functional and structural damage. The functional impairment is very much reversible, whereas the structural changes are mostly irreversible. Initially the studies related to antibody-mediated damage have been performed *in vitro* animals followed by human studies using functional magnetic resonance imaging (MRI), positron emission tomography (PET) scan, and histopathological specimens obtained on biopsy.

CLASSIFICATION

The revised International League against Epilepsy classification includes epilepsy due to autoimmune or inflammation under the etiology of epilepsies. These are further classified into epilepsies with antibodies against intracellular antigens (AICAs), epilepsies with antibodies against neuronal surface antigens, Rasmussen's encephalitis and fever induced refractory epilepsy in school-going children, etc.

AUTOIMMUNE ENCEPHALITIS

Autoimmune Encephalitis with Antibodies against Intracellular Antigens

This most common condition caused by AICA is paraneoplastic limbic encephalitis. Various tumors and the associated antibodies can cause similar clinical picture.

Limbic encephalitis is characterized by cognitive impairment, behavioral disturbances, seizures, and sleep disturbances. Seizures are the predominant manifestation in 70% of cases. These can be focal or secondary generalized. Status epilepticus is not uncommon. Paraneoplastic limbic encephalitis precedes diagnosis of cancer in about 50% of cases. Antibodies are directed against intracellular antigens shared by tumor cells and neurons. These onconeural antibodies are not directly pathogenic. The neurological involvement is due to cell-mediated immune reaction. A wide variety of such onconeural antibodies are recognized which include anti-Hu, anti-CV2/CRMP5, anti Ma2/Ta, anti-VGCC, anti-mGluR5 (Ophelia syndrome in Hodgkin lymphoma) antibodies.

In addition to classical features of limbic encephalitis, patients may also have widespread CNS and peripheral nervous system (PNS) involvement like encephalomyelitis, cerebellar degeneration and sensory neuronopathy. Hypothalamic dysfunction was seen in anti Ma2/Ta associated encephalitis.

In patients with paraneoplastic encephalitis, the immune system creates both a cytotoxic T-cell response and a humoral response against the same neoplastic antigens. Most likely, these antigen-specific activated T-cells cross the blood–brain barrier and attack the neurons that express these antigens in a major histocompatibility complex class I restricted manner. Such mechanisms have been shown in various animal models.

The MRI brain shows mesial temporal hyperintensities. Cerebrospinal fluid (CSF) may show mild elevation of protein and mild lymphocytic pleocytosis. The onconeural antibodies are detected in the serum of majority of patients but seronegativity is not uncommon. All patients should undergo screening for occult malignancy. Whole body 18F-fluoro-2-deoxyglucose (FDG)-PET is recommended to detect occult neoplasm. If initial PET scan is negative for malignancy, repeated screening every 6 months is recommended for up to 4 years. Onconeural antibodies can rarely occur in the absence of malignancy. Treatment includes treatment of underlying malignancy, which results in partial improvement. There is a poor response to immunotherapies.

Autoimmune Encephalitis with Antibodies to Neuronal Surface Antigens

This type of autoimmune encephalitis (AE) is more common and recently described. Most of them are nonparaneoplastic and have a good response to immunotherapy. Table 1 illustrates the differences between these and the AE due to antibodies against intracellular antigens.

Voltage-gated Potassium Channel Complex Antibody Limbic Encephalitis

The VGKC complex antibody encephalitis is the most common type of AE which is usually not associated with a tumor. These antibodies are directed to proteins that are associated with the VGKC complex, rather than with the VGKC itself. Until now, three different target proteins have been recognized: contactin-associated protein-like 2 (Caspr2), leucine-rich

TABLE 1: Depicts the differences between the two major types of autoimmune encephalitis

	Classical paraneoplastic CNS syndrome associated with onconeural antibodies	CNS syndrome associated with neuronal surface antibodies
Main syndromes	• Cerebellar degeneration • Encephalomyelitis • Limbic encephalitis • Brain stem encephalitis	• Limbic encephalitis • Monan's syndrome • NMDAR Ab encephalitis • PERM (progressive encephalomyelitis with rigidity and myoclonus) • Cerebellar ataxia
Age range (years) and sex	Mainly adults (40–70), both genders (PCD more frequent in women)	NMDAR-Ab encephalitis common in children and young women
Antibodies commonly detected or recently reported	Antibodies against intracellular antigens or PNS-related onconeural antibodies (Hu, Yo, Ri, Ma2, Cv2 / CRMP5, amphiphysin, SoxI/2)	Antibodies to VGKC complex antigens (LGLI or CASPR2), NMDAR, AMIPAR, GABA1R, GlyR, VGCC Ab, mGluR1, mGluR5
Immunopatho-genesis	Antibodies are markers for the tumor and are not likely to be pathogenic. T cell cytotoxicity is the proposed pathogenic mechanism	Autoantibody mediated, probably down regulation of target antigen but may be complement mediated damage in same conditions. Limited data variable T cells. B cells and plasma cell infiltrates but less intense than in patient with paraneoplastic disease
Immunotherapy and outcome	Not usually effective. Poor, improvement or stabilization related mainly to tumor treatment	Generally effective. Variable but generally good; possible spontaneous remission
Tumors	Some antibodies usually indicates the presence of particular tumor type. SCLC, breast, ovary, testicular	No tumor found in many cases, particularly LE associated with LGLI - Ab. NMDA encephalitis associated with ovarian Teratoma. mGlur5 Ab with Hodgkins disease
Relationship between antibody and disease	Antibody usually indicated the presence of particular tumor type	Antibody presence does not indicate if a case as paraneoplastic

glioma inactivated 1 (LGI1) and the protein contactin-2. In most cases, the antibodies are directed against LGI1.

The LGI1 antibodies are associated with a typical course of limbic encephalitis, characterized by memory loss, confusion, behavioral change, and seizures. The Caspr2 antibodies are more commonly associated with involvement at the level of neuromuscular junction causing neuromyotonia or Issac syndrome. In few cases, there is combination of CNS and PNS involvement called as Morvan's syndrome. In addition, some cases with Caspr2 antibodies present with cerebellar ataxia.

Animal studies in rats have shown that there is a binding of LGI1 antibodies to the hippocampal neuropil. Domestic cats serve as a new model for this disease as they suffer from epilepsy with orofacial seizures that show some similarities to the dystonic faciobrachial seizures in patients when LGI1 antibodies are transferred to them and thus serve as the new model for this disease. The LGI1 antibodies induces complement activation and cause neuronal cell death resulting in hippocampal atrophy.

This type of encephalitis (VGKC complex related) is more common in men and occurs mostly after the age of 40 years. Seizures occur in 80% of cases and usually are focal with impaired awareness and are secondary generalized. Ictal autonomic manifestations, like piloerection, have been reported. Hyponatremia (less than 130 mEq/L) occurs in 30–60% of the cases due to the syndrome of inappropriate secretion of antidiuretic hormone.

A subgroup of LGI1 antibodies has been recognized which presents with a peculiar faciobrachial dystonic seizure (FBDS) during their prodromal phase before the development of cognitive disturbances. These seizures occur up to hundreds of times per day, and are characterized by brief tonic contraction of the arm and face, either on one side or, more commonly, alternating between both sides. Electroencephalography (EEG) changes during FBDS most often consist of diffuse attenuation or bursts of slow waves. Brain FDG-PET may show hypermetabolism in the basal ganglia. There is a controversy over whether FBDS are truly epileptic seizures or a kind of movement disorder. It highlights the traditional border zones between epilepsy and movement disorders. Imaging studies suggest that a simultaneous involvement of frontal cortex and basal ganglia contribute to this type of event. These FBDS do not respond to AEDs. Though immunomodulatory treatment is efficacious and might prevent the occurrence of cognitive impairment.

Cerebrospinal fluid analysis is most often normal. Brain MRI is abnormal in half the cases, commonly showing hyperintensities in the mesial temporal lobes and sometimes basal ganglia. Most patients with anti-VGKC complex antibodies are nonparaneoplastic and do not have an associated neoplasm. Treatment with steroids, intravenous immunoglobulin (IVIg), or plasma exchange is efficacious, and most patients make a full recovery. Clinical improvement is accompanied by the decreasing antibody titer in the serum.

Autoimmune Encephalitis with Antibodies against NMDA Receptor

Anti-NMDA receptor encephalitis was first described in patients with paraneoplastic encephalitis resulting from ovarian teratomas. Some years later, it was shown that the antibodies reacted with the NR1 subunit of the NMDA receptor, and the NMDA receptor encephalitis also could be found in the absence of a tumor.

This type of encephalitis is common in young adult females. It often begins with a nonspecific febrile illness. A few weeks later, patients present with behavioral changes, delusions, hallucinations, and anxiety. Short-term memory loss and seizures usually occur at this stage. Seizures are most commonly of the generalized tonic-clonic type, but occasionally focal seizures can also occur. Male patients tend to present more frequently with seizures at onset than female patients. Status epilepticus can occur and can be refractory. The encephalopathy then progresses to a severe catatonic stage, during which patients alternate between periods of akinesia and periods of violent agitation. At this stage, most patients develop typical orofacial dyskinesia, dysautonomia and hypoventilation, requiring prolonged ventilator support.

Typically, in many cases, the EEG shows generalized delta activity, which is often rhythmic. At least 50% of patients exhibit a disease-specific pattern of generalized rhythmic delta activity with superimposed beta or even gamma activity, termed extreme delta brushes (EDB) because of their resemblance to the delta brushes of neonates. Figure 1 depicts an EEG showing EDB in a case of anti-NMDA receptor encephalitis.

Cerebrospinal fluid analysis is abnormal in more than majority of cases (90%) commonly showing a mild lymphocytosis. Brain MRI shows T2/fluid-attenuated inversion recovery (FLAIR) hyperintensities in neocortical areas or occasionally in the mesial temporal lobes, basal ganglia, or brainstem. Cortical atrophy usually develops with time.

Approximately half of the female patients have an ovarian teratoma. Pelvic MRI is more sensitive than computed tomography (CT) scan and ultrasound, but the tumor can be microscopic and escape imaging techniques. Treatment includes tumor resection and immune therapy.

First-line treatment is with steroids or IVIg which often fails (more than 50%), and second-line therapy with cyclophosphamide or rituximab is required. Most patients ultimately respond, and many regain near-normal functional status. Early treatment and response to first-line therapy are good prognostic indicators. It may take up to 2 years and even longer before patients recover fully from anti-NMDA receptor encephalitis. Long-term deficits are common in the form of sleep disturbances and executive dysfunction. Figure 1 shows an illustrative case showing the problems faced in the management.

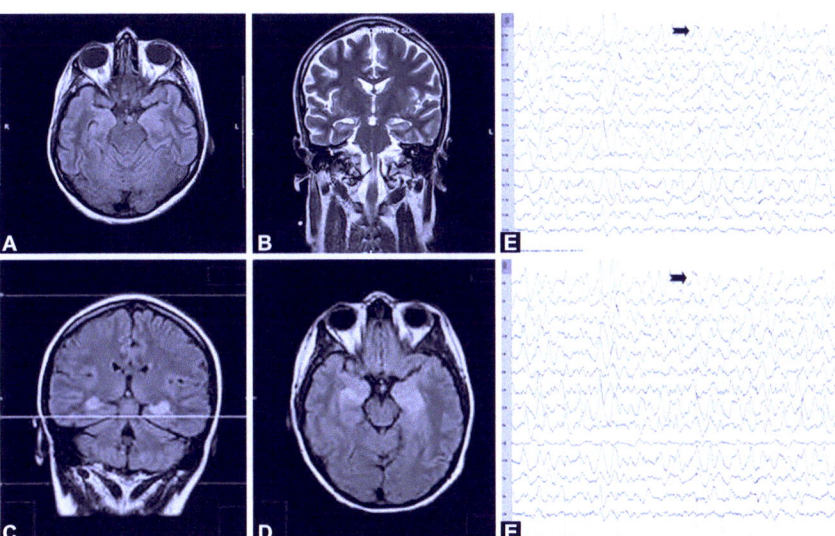

Note: She was also having a small ovarian teratoma but could not be operated in view of poor general condition.

FIG. 1: A 23-year-old lady presented with fever followed by seizures and abnormal behavior. Her initial MRI Brain **A** and **B,** was normal. She was diagnosed as viral meningoencephalitis and treated empirically with acyclovir and antipsychotics. She developed orofacial dyskinesias which were thought to be drug induced and antipsychotics were stopped. Slowly she became mute, developed dysautonomia and hypoventilation for which she was intubated and brought to our hospital. Repeat MRI Brain **C** and **D,** showed bilateral mesial temporal hyperintensities and EEG **E,** demonstrated extreme delta brushes (solid arrow). A diagnosis of NMDA receptor encephalitis was made. Serum and CSF both were showing NMDA receptor antibodies. Patient was treated with steroids and IVIG without any clinical response. Second line immunotherapy with rituximab was given. Patient succumbed to the illness secondary to severe respiratory tract infection. *(For color version, see plate 1)*

An *in vitro* study by Hughes et al. demonstrated that this antibody cross-links NMDA receptors, thereby causing their internalization into the cell. The internalization of the NMDA receptor results in a reversible hypofunction without destruction of the nerve cells or synapses. This also affects the long-term potentiation required for episodic memory. The above reasons explain the psychotic features and anterograde amnesia which is so characteristic of the disease. The frequent occurrence of seizures and even status epilepticus, is not easily explained by an NMDA receptor hypofunction, as paradoxically NMDA receptor blockers like ketamine exert an antiepileptic effect and are used in status epilepticus. Both *in vivo* and *in vitro* studies have shown increased extracellular glutamate concentrations in patients with NMDA receptor encephalitis explaining the pathogenesis.

Anti-gamma Amino Butyric Acid B Receptor Encephalitis

Only few cases are reported in the literature. Almost all presented with limbic encephalitis and prominent seizures or status epilepticus. Gamma amino butyric acid-B (GABA-B) receptor antibodies may be absent from patients' serum and detected only in the CSF. Brain MRI demonstrates hyperintensities in the mesial temporal lobes and CSF analysis may reveal pleocytosis.

Most common neoplasm associated is small cell lung carcinoma. Approximately 20–30% of patients have onconeural antibodies (SOX1, Hu, amphiphysin). Patients usually tend to have other autoimmune diseases (including type 1 diabetes mellitus, idiopathic thrombocytopenia, and thyroiditis). Most patients respond at least partially to immune treatment and tumor removal, and some make a full recovery.

Gamma Amino Butyric Acid-A Receptor Antibody Encephalitis

This is also rare. Clinical presentation is variable, although it is consistent with limbic encephalitis in some patients. Refractory status epilepticus with multifocal cortical MRI abnormalities have also been described. Similar to patients with GABA-B receptor antibodies, these cases also have associated autoimmune disease and other neuronal surface antigens. Half of the patients who received immune therapies responded at least partially.

AMPA Receptor Antibody Encephalitis

The antibodies against glutamate receptor 1 or 2 subunit of the alpha-amino-3-hydroxy-5-methyl-4-isoxazole-propionic acid (AMPA) receptor have been described. This is seen in middle-aged women. They often have prominent psychiatric symptoms. Association with small cell lung carcinoma is common. Response to treatment (immune therapy with or without tumor removal) is good but most experience recurrent relapses even after tumor removal.

Glycine Receptor Antibody Encephalitis

These have been described in association with stiff person syndrome and progressive encephalomyelitis with rigidity and myoclonus, but a few cases of limbic encephalitis with seizures and status epilepticus are also described. An association with neoplasm is rare.

Limbic Encephalitis Associated with GAD-65 Antibodies

Antibodies against glutamic acid decarboxylase-65 (GAD-65) are directly pathogenic and trigger cellular inflammatory response. They are found in patients with stiff person syndrome, autoimmune cerebellar degeneration and in some patients with type 1 diabetes mellitus. Limbic encephalitis associated with antibodies against GAD-65 is seen in young females. The clinical features of encephalitis are very similar to limbic encephalitis associated with VGKC antibodies but have a more chronic course. Antibodies can be detected in serum and CSF. Few patients showed association with small cell lung cancer. There is poor response to immunotherapy.

Metabotropic Glutamate Receptor 5 Antibody–Mediated Encephalitis

Antibodies to metabotropic glutamate receptor 5 (mGluR5), a metabotropic glutamate receptor, have been reported in two patients with Hodgkin lymphoma and encephalitis, termed Ophelia syndrome. Symptoms are usually consistent with limbic encephalitis and they tend to have repeated seizures. The MRI shows more extensive radiologic involvement, including parietal and occipital cortex.

Dipeptidyl Peptidase-Like Protein-6 Antibody-Mediated Encephalitis

Dipeptidyl-peptidase-like protein-6 (DPPX) is a cell surface auxiliary subunit of the Kv4.2 potassium channels. It is expressed in the hippocampus and cerebellum and also in the myenteric plexus. Antibodies to DPPX can produce a protracted encephalitis characterized by nervous hyperexcitability resulting in agitation, myoclonus, tremor, and seizures along with frequent diarrhea at symptom onset.

Table 2 summarizes the clinical presentation of AE and the various antibodies associated with it.

Rasmussen's Encephalitis

Rasmussen's encephalitis is a rare disorder, characterized by unilateral inflammation of the cerebral cortex, drug-resistant focal epilepsy, and progressive neurological and cognitive impairment. There are descriptions of bilateral, lobar and even brainstem involvement.

Rasmussen's encephalitis was previously thought to be due to antibodies against GluR3 but recent studies have shown that it is driven by a T-cell response to one or more antigenic epitopes, with an additional contribution by autoantibodies.

It is common in children and young adults. The disease course involves three stages. A prodromal stage characterized by mild hemiparesis or infrequent seizure, an acute stage which is characterized by frequent seizures, often epilepsia partialis continua, progressive hemiparesis, hemianopia, cognitive deterioration, and aphasia (if dominant hemisphere affected); a residual stage characterized by permanent neurological deficits and continuous seizures. Diagnosis is based on clinical, EEG and radiological criteria.

Treatment with antiseizure medications is usually disappointing. Immunotherapy (steroids or IVIg) are effective if started early in the course of illness. Intravenous immunoglobulin is supposed to be more effective in adult Rasmussen's encephalitis which usually has more protracted course.

In later stages, seizure control is effectively achieved in about 85% of patients with surgical interventions like hemispherectomy or hemispherotomy but the benefit comes at the cost of significant neurological deficit. Language may be severely impaired in case of dominant hemisphere involvement. In such cases, immunotherapy with steroids, IVIg, and plasma exchange is the preferred option. Other drugs tried in the disease were tacrolimus, natalizumab, and rituximab. Box 1 shows the diagnostic criteria for Rasmussen's encephalitis.

TABLE 2: Major clinical presentations of autoimmune encephalitis and their associated antibodies, neoplasms and response to treatment

Syndrome	Antibodies	Particular clinical features	Possible tumors	Immunotherapy response
NMDAR-Ab encephalitis	NMDAR	Dystonic movements, psychiatric presentation in young women. Epilepsy and abnormal movements more frequent at onset in children	• Ovarian teratoma • Rare in children. Up to 50% after age 18 years	Yes
Limbic encephalitis	LGLI CASPR2 (<10%)	Male predominance, hyponatremia, faciobrachial dystonic seizures, myoclonus	Rare with LGL1-Ab, thymoma in some with CASPR2-Ab	Yes
	AMPAR	Possible isolated psychiatric symptoms	70% (lung, breast, thymus)	Yes, frequent relapses
	GABABR	Prominent seizures	60% (SCLC)	Yes
	mGluR5	Ophelia syndrome	Hodgkin lymphoma	Unknown
Morvan's syndrome	CASPR2	Encephalopathy, peripheral nerve hyperexcitability, dysautonomia	Thymoma	Yes
PERM (paraneoplastic encephalomyelitis with rigidity and myoclonus)	GlyR	Encephalomyelitis with myoclonus, rigidity and brainstems signs	Thymoma	Yes
Cerebellar ataxia	VGCC	Possible co-existence of LEMS	SCLC	Poor
	mGluRl	Remote history of Hodgkin lymphoma	Hodgkin lymphoma	Yes

SYNDROMES OF DE NOVO FEBRILE ILLNESS-RELATED REFRACTORY SEIZURES AND STATUS EPILEPTICUS

These syndromes have received various names, including new-onset refractory status epilepticus (NORSE), febrile infection-related epilepsy syndrome (FIRES), and acute encephalitis with refractory repetitive partial seizures (AERRPS). These syndromes

> **Box 1: Clinical criteria for diagnosis of Rasmussens encephalitis**
>
> **Part A (all three)**
> - Clinical: Focal seizures (with or without epilepsia partialis continua) and unilateral deficits
> - MRI: Unihemispheric focal cortical atrophy and at least one of the following:
>   - Gray or white matter T2/FLAIR hyperintense signal
>   - Hyperintense signal or atrophy of the ipsilateral caudate head
> - EEG: Unilateral slowing with or without epileptiform activity and unilateral seizure onset
>
> **Part B (two of three)**
> - Clinical: Epilepsia partialis continua or progressive unilateral cortical deficits
> - MRI: Progressive unihemispheric focal cortical atrophy
> - Histopathology: T-cell dominated encephalitis with activated microglial cells typically, but not necessarily, forming nodules and reactive astrogliosis; numerous parenchyma macrophages

are characterized by the sudden onset of frequent seizures and status epilepticus in an otherwise healthy individual, often bilateral or multifocal. Status epilepticus is usually highly refractory and can last for weeks. Mortality is high, and most survivors develop pharmacoresistant epilepsy. The CSF analysis and MRI often show changes suggestive of encephalitis but usually no causative virus or antibody is isolated. Long-term cognitive impairment is frequent but some patients make a full recovery. The cause of these syndromes is currently unknown. Recent studies have shown high levels of proconvulsant cytokines in the CSF of children with this disease. Treatment with antiepileptics and anesthetics is often disappointing, but immune therapies and the ketogenic diet occasionally prove to be effective.

SEIZURES IN PATIENTS WITH OTHER AUTOIMMUNE AND INFLAMMATORY DISORDERS OF THE CNS

There is 2–3 times increased risk of seizures in patients with multiple sclerosis compared with general population. The mechanism is not completely understood. Seizures occur in two-thirds of patients with severe acute disseminated encephalomyelitis. Epilepsia partialis continua and nonconvulsive status epilepticus can occur but are infrequent manifestations. Seizures can occur in 20% of patients with CNS vasculitis. There is 2–9-fold increased risk of seizures in patients with systemic autoimmune diseases. Most common systemic autoimmune diseases associated with seizures are systemic lupus erythematosus (SLE), antiphospholipid antibodies and type 1 diabetes mellitus. The mechanism of seizures is not only autoimmune process, but other mechanisms like ischemic injury, organ failure, drug toxicity, opportunistic infections, and coexistence of autoantibodies against neuronal surface antigens also play a role.

In SLE, 15% of patients will have seizures and presence of seizures is one of the diagnostic criteria for SLE. Children and patients with antiphospholipid antibodies are at increased risk of seizures.

Seizures occur in about two-third cases of Hashimoto's encephalopathy, which is now called steroid responsive encephalopathy with autoimmune thyroiditis. Patients have high titers of antibodies against thyroperoxidase or thyroglobulin. Dramatic response to steroids is seen in this condition.

Seizures also occur in Sjogren's syndrome, Behcet's disease, sarcoidosis, and Wegener's granulomatosis. A rare form of occipital epilepsy with occipital cerebral calcification has been reported in patients with celiac disease in southern Europe and South America.

ANTIBODIES IN PATIENTS WITH ISOLATED CHRONIC EPILEPSY

Some patients continue to have seizures after a treated episode of AE. In such cases, seizures are a result of postencephalitic irreversible brain injury and they do not require immunotherapy. These patients qualify for the diagnosis of epilepsy. Autoimmune limbic encephalitis may present as temporal lobe epilepsy with hippocampal sclerosis. These patients tend to have a higher seizure frequency, memory impairment, and bilateral hippocampal involvement.

Some patients with epilepsy have antibodies to neuronal surface antigens, but the significance of this finding is still not clear. A minority of patients with epilepsy and VGKC complex and GAD-65 antibodies appear to have a mild form of limbic encephalitis, in which seizures predominate. Clinical clues to the diagnosis of autoimmune epilepsy are summarized in Box 2.

Box 2: Clinical clues for the suspicion of autoimmune epilepsy

Historical data
- Personal or family history of autoimmne disorders or seropositivity for organ-specific (e.g. thyroid) or non-organ specific autoantibodies (e.g. rheumatoid arthritis)
- Recent or past history of neoplasia

Clinical data
- Acute to sub-acute onset of symptoms(weeks to months)
- Rapidly progressive or fluctuating course with multifocal neurological signs and symptoms
- Presence of cognitive and memory impairment, psychiatric disturbances, autonomic and sleep-related dysfunction, myoclonus and movement disorders including oro-facial dyskinesias

Seizure characteristics
- High seizure frequency
- New onset status epilepticus
- Multifocal seizures or multiple semiologies
- Faciobrachial dystonic seizures
- Adult onset temporal lobe epilepsy with high frequency of seizures and no obvious cause
- Antiepileptic drug resistance

Investigations
- Mesial temporal or parenchymal hyperintensity in MRI
- Elevated proteins, pleocytosis (>5 cells/mm^3). Oligoclonal bands, elevated IgG index or elevated neopterin (>30 nm) in CSF
- "Extreme delta brush" in EEG rhythmic delta waves at 1–3/s with superimposed burst of rhythmic 20–30/s β activity
- Hypermetabolism in positron emission tomography
- Inflammatory neuropathology on biopsy

INTERPRETATION OF ANTIBODY TESTING IN AUTOIMMUNE ENCEPHALITIS

Testing of antibodies in suspected cases should be done in both serum and CSF. A positive CSF finding with a negative serum suggests intrathecal synthesis, which is especially seen with NMDA receptor antibodies. A positive serum with a negative CSF usually indicates a false-positive result, although this can be seen with LGI1 and Caspr2 antibodies. A negative antibody test does not rule out AE. Figure 2 illustrates a case of AE, which was negative for antibody testing.

TREATMENT

Intravenous steroids, IVIg and plasma exchange are the first-line treatment options. When compared to other autoimmune diseases like myasthenia gravis, the response to treatment with these immunotherapies is slow and less effective probably due to the presence of intrathecal antibodies or presence of an associated cellular immune response and delayed recovery of the more complex CNS. Patients with LGI1 encephalitis (characterized by infrequent intrathecal antibody synthesis) respond faster than patients with NMDA receptor encephalitis (characterized by very frequent intrathecal antibody synthesis). In patients who do not respond to first-line treatment, rituximab or cyclophosphamide can be used. In case of paraneoplastic limbic encephalitis, removal of the underlying neoplasm is necessary.

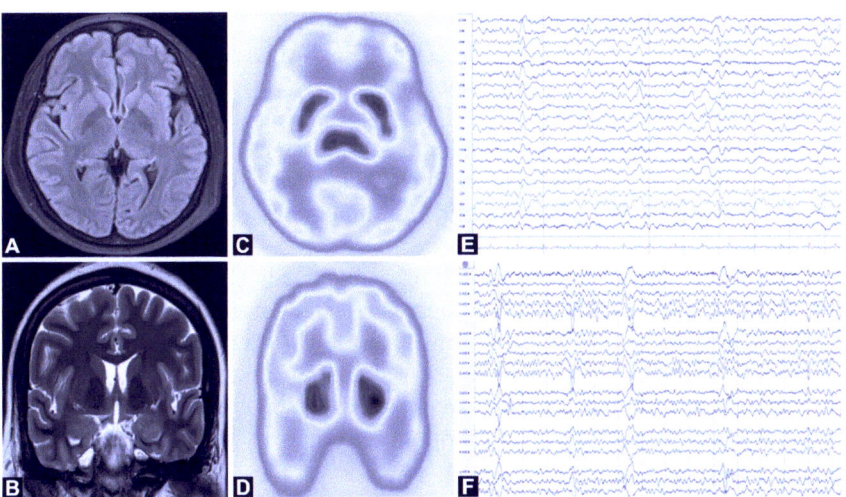

FIG. 2: A 38-year-old lady presented with low grade fever for 2 weeks followed by psychiatric disturbances in the form of delusions and hallucinations, 3 episodes of GTCS and infrequent myoclonus. Neurological examination revealed impaired memory and executive dysfunction. MRI Brain **A** and **B,** was normal. CT PET scan **C** and **D,** showed Bilateral basal ganglionic hypermetabolism. EEG **E** and **F,** revealed diffuse theta to delta range slowing. CSF analysis was normal. Serum and CSF analysis for antibodies (onconeural and ANSA) were negative. She was emperically treated with steroids with which she had a dramatic improvement. A diagnosis of Autoimmune encephalitis was made in the absence of antibodies. *(For color version, see plate 2)*

CONCLUSION

Autoimmune epilepsy is a new and exciting concept. Clinicians should have a high level of suspicion when dealing with refractory epilepsy, especially of recent onset and where the etiology could not be established by routine investigations, and look for serum autoantibodies. Early initiation of immunotherapy is vital for better outcome and may also be tried if the clinical suspicion is high even if the antibody screening is negative.

TAKE HOME MESSAGES

- Paraneoplastic limbic encephalitis presents with memory loss, seizures, and behavioral and sleep disturbances. The condition can occur in isolation or in association with signs of widespread neurologic involvement
- A diagnosis of limbic encephalitis should prompt thorough and repeated investigations for an occult malignancy. Positron emission tomography is superior to CT for the detection of small lesions
- The most common antigen recognized by VGKC is leucine-rich, glioma inactivated 1 (LGI1). The syndrome is one of limbic encephalitis in middle-aged men, often associated with hyponatremia
- Faciobrachial dystonic seizures consist of brief tonic contractions of the face and arm that occur exclusively in association with LGI1 antibodies and precede the manifestations of limbic encephalitis
- N-methyl-D-aspartate receptor antibodies are the most commonly identified antibodies directed to neuronal surface antigens. The syndrome is one of behavioral and psychiatric manifestations, followed by a severe catatonic phase with movement disorders and autonomic instability
- Extreme delta brushes are a specific EEG feature of NMDA receptor encephalitis. They are encountered in approximately half of the cases
- Antibodies directed toward neuronal surface antigens, AMPA, GABA-A receptor, GABA-B receptor, and glycine receptors have been identified but need to be further characterized. They are associated with limbic encephalitis or neocortical encephalitis with seizures and status epilepticus and are sometimes associated with neoplasms or autoimmune diseases
- Rasmussen's encephalitis presents with refractory focal epilepsy, neurologic decline, and progressive cortical atrophy. Antibodies directed toward the glutamate receptor 3 are no longer thought to be causal and T-cell mediated immunity is incriminated. Treatment includes antiseizure medications, immune therapy, and often surgery
- Uncommon cases of currently cryptogenic refractory status epilepticus, termed FIRES and NORSE in adults, may have an autoimmune origin.

SUGGESTED READINGS

1. Becker EB, Zuliani L, Pettingill R, et al. Contactin-associated protein-2 antibodies in non-paraneoplastic cerebellar ataxia. J Neurol Neurosurg Psychiatry. 2012;83;437-40.
2. Berg AT, Berkovic SF, Brodie MJ, et al. Revised terminology and concepts for organization of seizures and epilepsies: Report of the ILAE Commission on Classification and Terminology, 2005-2009. Epilepsia. 2010;51(4):676-85.
3. Bien CG, Granata T, Antozzi C, et al. Pathogenesis, diagnosis and treatment of Rasmussen encephalitis: A European consensus statement. Brain. 2005;128(Pt 3):454-71.

4. Bien CG, Scheffer IE. Autoantibodies and epilepsy. Epilepsia. 2011;52(Suppl 3):18-22.
5. Bien CG, Vincent A, Barnett MH, et al. Immunopathology of autoantibody-associated encephalitides: Clues for pathogenesis. Brain. 2012;135;1622-38.
6. Boesebeck F, Schwarz O, Dohmen B, et al. Faciobrachial dystonic seizures arise from cortico-subcortical abnormal brain areas. J Neurol. 2013;260:1684-6.
7. Boronat A, Gelfand JM, Gresa-Arribas N, et al. Encephalitis and antibodies to dipeptidyl-peptidase-like protein-6, a subunit of Kv4.2 potassium channels. Ann Neurol. 2013;73(1):120-8.
8. Brain L, Jellinek EH, Ball K. Hashimoto's disease and encephalopathy. Lancet. 1966;2(7462):51-4.
9. Brenner T, Sills GJ, Hart Y, et al. Prevalence of neurologic autoantibodies in cohorts of patients with new and established epilepsy. Epilepsia. 2013;54(6):102-35.
10. Carvajal-González A, Leite MI, Waters P, et al. Glycine receptor antibodies in PERM and related syndromes: Characteristics, clinical features and outcomes. Brain. 2014;137(pt 8):217-92.
11. Chan D, Henley SM, Rossor MN, et al. Extensive and temporally ungraded retrograde amnesia in encephalitis associated with antibodies to voltage-gated potassium channels. Arch Neurol. 2007;64;404-10.
12. Dalmau J, Gleichman AJ, Hughes EG, et al. Anti-NMDA-receptor encephalitis: Case series and analysis of the effects of antibodies. Lancet Neurol. 2008;7:1091-8.
13. Dalmau J, Rosenfeld MR. Paraneoplastic syndromes of the CNS. Lancet Neurol. 2008;7(4):327-40.
14. Finke C, Kopp UA, Scheel M, et al. Functional and structural brain changes in anti-N-methyl-D-aspartate receptor encephalitis. Ann Neurol. 2013;74(2):284-96.
15. Giometto B, Grisold W, Vitaliani R, et al. Paraneoplastic neurologic syndrome in the PNS Euronetwork database: A European study from 20 centers. Arch Neurol. 2010;67:330-13.
16. Graus F, Boronat A, Xifro X, et al. The expanding clinical profile of anti-AMPA receptor encephalitis. Neurology. 2010;74(10):857-9.
17. Hughes EG, Peng X, Gleichman AJ, et al. Cellular and synaptic mechanisms of anti-NMDA receptor encephalitis. J Neurosci. 2010;30;5866-75.
18. Höftberger R, Titulaer MJ, Sabater L, et al. Encephalitis and GABAB receptor antibodies: Novel findings in a new case series of 20 patients. Neurology. 2013;81(17):150-6.
19. Irani SR, Alexander S, Waters P, et al. Antibodies to Kv1 potassium channel-complex proteins leucine-rich, glioma inactivated 1 protein and contactin-associated protein-2 in limbic encephalitis, Morvan's syndrome and acquired neuromyotonia. Brain. 2010;133;2734-48.
20. Irani SR, Bien CG, Lang B. Autoimmune epilepsies. Curr Opin Neurol. 2011;24(2):146-53.
21. Irani SR, Stagg CJ, Schott JM, et al. Faciobrachial dystonic seizures: The influence of immunotherapy on seizure control and prevention of cognitive impairment in a broadening phenotype. Brain. 2013;136:3151-62.
22. Ismail FY, Kossoff EH. AERRPS, DESC, NORSE FIRES: Multi-labeling or distinct epileptic entities? Epilepsia. 2011;52(11):e18-9.
23. Lalic T, Pettingill P, Vincent A, et al. Human limbic encephalitis serum enhances hippocampal mossy fiber-CA3 pyramidal cell synaptic transmission. Epilepsia. 2011;52;121-31.
24. Lancaster E, Lai M, Peng X, et al. Antibodies to the GABA(B) receptor in limbic encephalitis with seizures: Case series and characterization of the antigen. Lancet Neurol. 2010;9(1):67-76.
25. Lancaster E, Martinez-Hernandez E, Titulaer MJ, et al. Antibodies to metabotropic glutamate receptor 5 in the Ophelia syndrome. Neurology. 2011;77(18):1698-1701.
26. Pakozdy A, Gruber A, Kneissl S, et al. Complex partial cluster seizures in cats with orofacial involvement. J Feline Med Surg. 2011;13:687-93.
27. Pellkofer H, Schubart AS, Hoftberger R, et al. Modelling paraneoplastic CNS disease: T-cells specific for the onconeuronal antigen PNMA1 mediate autoimmune encephalomyelitis in the rat. Brain. 2004;127:1822-30.
28. Pettingill P, Kramer HB, Coebergh JA, et al. Antibodies to GABAA receptor !1 and ,2 subunits: Clinical and serologic characterization. Neurology. 2015;84(12):123-41.
29. Quek AM, Britton JW, McKeon A, et al. Autoimmune epilepsy: Clinical characteristics and response to immunotherapy. Arch Neurol 2012;69;582-93.
30. Saiz A, Blanco Y, Sabater L, et al. Spectrum of neurological syndromes associated with glutamic acid decarboxylase antibodies: Diagnostic clues for this association. Brain. 2008;131(pt 10):255-63.

31. Sakuma H, Tanuma N, Kuki I, et al. Intrathecal overproduction of proinflammatory cytokines and chemokines in febrile infection-related refractory status epilepticus. J Neurol Neurosurg Psychiatry. 2015;86(7):820-2.
32. Solimena M, Folli F, Denis Donini S, et al. Autoantibodies to glutamic acid decarboxylase in a patient with stiff-man syndrome, epilepsy, and type I diabetes mellitus. N Engl J Med. 1988;318;1012-20.
33. Vincent A, Buckley C, Schott JM, et al. Potassium channel antibody- associated encephalopathy: A potentially immunotherapy-responsive form of limbic encephalitis. Brain. 2004;127;701-12.
34. Vincent A, Irani SR, Lang B. The growing recognition of immunotherapy-responsive seizure disorders with autoantibodies to specific neuronal proteins. Curr Opin Neurol. 2010;23(2):144–150.
35. Zuliani L, Graus F, Giometto B, et al. Central nervous system neuronal surface antibody associated syndromes: Review and guidelines for recognition. J Neurol Neurosurg Psychiatry. 2012;83(6): 638-45.

CHAPTER 7

Autoimmune Movement Disorders

Syam Krishnan Nair

INTRODUCTION

Movement disorders result from a variety of pathogenetic mechanisms affecting the components of basal ganglia circuits or their connections. Less frequently, movement disorders could arise from more peripheral mechanisms. Autoimmunity is being increasingly recognized as a cause of movement disorders in children as well as adults. As autoimmune movement disorders are relatively uncommon, a high index of suspicion in cases with phenomenology and temporal evolution concordant with autoimmune disorders is needed to order targeted investigations, arrive at a diagnosis and initiate timely management. This review discusses various autoimmune movement disorder clinical syndromes and provides an overview of diagnostic approach and management.

GENERAL APPROACH TO MOVEMENT DISORDERS

Movement disorders are those conditions which manifest as involuntary or "unvoluntary" (lying in between the two extremes of voluntary and completely involuntary) movements or disturbances in the amplitude, velocity, or precision of voluntary movements without weakness or paralysis of the involved musculature. Tics and stereotypies, which are not suppressible fully but possess a volitional component, are examples of unvoluntary movements. Ataxia which results primarily from disturbances in cerebellar or proprioceptive function, though covered by the definition, is often considered as a separate clinical entity.

Movement disorders can be classified broadly into two groups—hypokinetic or bradykinetic disorders (characterized by reduced amplitude and speed of voluntary movements) and hyperkinetic or dyskinetic disorders (characterized by the presence of abnormal, involuntary movements). Hypokinesia (reduced amplitude of movements) and bradykinesia (reduced speed) are closely related and often accompanied by increased muscle tone (rigidity), and sometimes rest tremor, and this combination is denoted as "Parkinsonism". Parkinsonism by definition needs bradykinesia as a mandatory feature along with at least one more among rigidity and rest tremor. Though postural instability is also seen in many patients with Parkinsonism, it is not currently considered as a cardinal feature and not taken into account in defining Parkinsonism. Hypokinetic and hyperkinetic manifestations coexist in several basal ganglia disorders, like Parkinson's disease where rigidity and bradykinesia occur along with rest tremor (which is a hyperkinetic movement disorder) in many patients.

Movement disorders could result from a variety of insults to the basal ganglia and its connections like genetic (heredodegenerative or inherited metabolic), degenerative, inflammatory, neoplastic, toxic, traumatic, or vascular. Similar to movement disorders due to other causes, the first step in the diagnosis of a suspected autoimmune movement disorder is the proper identification of the movement disorder phenomenology. A phenomenological classification of hyperkinetic movement disorders is presented in Table 1. Movement disorders arising from autoimmunity may have any of these phenomenologies in isolation, may occur as a combination of multiple phenomenologies or could be combined with other neurologic (nonmovement disorder) or systemic manifestations.

AUTOIMMUNE MOVEMENT DISORDERS

Movement disorders from autoimmune causes occur both in children and in adults. For practical purposes, these can be classified into parainfectious, paraneoplastic, idiopathic

TABLE 1: Hyperkinetic movement disorders and their phenomenological characteristics

Movement disorder	Characteristics
Dystonia	A movement disorder, characterized by sustained or intermittent muscle contractions causing abnormal and often repetitive movements, postures or both. The movements are generally patterned and twisting. Could be associated with tremor (dystonic tremor). Could occur at rest or during action; dystonia at rest is generally worsened by voluntary action
Tremor	Rhythmic involuntary sinusoidal alternating movements of a body part. Can be further classified into tremor occurring at rest or with action. Action tremor could be postural (when the affected body part is held against gravity), kinetic (during movement), intention (during movement, but worsens toward reaching the target), task specific (occur during specific tasks only, like writing) and isometric (during voluntary muscle contractions against a fixed resistance). Combination of rest, postural and kinetic tremor of large amplitude can be seen in midbrain lesions ("Rubral tremor" or "Holmes tremor")
Chorea	Abrupt, unpredictable and nonrhythmic (do not recur at regular intervals) involuntary movements resulting from a continual, random "flow" of muscle contractions. Gives a "fidgety" or, when more severe, dancing appearance
Myoclonus	The fastest involuntary movement. Sudden, brief, jerky, and electric shock-like in character. Named as positive myoclonus when caused by muscle contraction, or negative myoclonus when it results from a transient loss of muscle tone. Can result from cortical or subcortical mechanisms. Can mimic tremor when it is repetitive and rhythmic (recurring at regular and short intervals)
Tics	An "unvoluntary" movement (it is temporarily suppressible by the patient; see text) preceded by a mounting urge ("sensory trick") to perform the movement and relieved by performance of the movement. Could be simple, like eye blinking or shoulder shrugging, or more complex. Tics are stereotyped and repetitive, but generally not rhythmic
Stereotypies	Similar to tics, in that they are unvoluntary. However, these are more complex, patterned and ritualistic. They are less paroxysmal and repeated in a continual fashion. Often seen in patients who are autistic and cognitively impaired; the sensory component seen in tics is absent

and those associated with systemic autoimmune disorders. Some of the autoimmune movement disorder syndromes could occur both as a parainfectious or as a paraneoplastic manifestation. In addition, inflammatory disorders of the central nervous system (CNS) of autoimmune etiology like multiple sclerosis, acute disseminated encephalomyelitis (ADEM), and CNS vasculitis can result in structural damage presenting as movement disorder manifestations (Holmes tremor in multiple sclerosis, dystonia as a sequela of putaminal or thalamic involvement by ADEM, etc.). These will not be further considered in this review. Autoimmune cerebellar disorders and involuntary movements from peripheral nerve hyperexcitability and muscle disorders also will not be discussed and are addressed in the other relevant sections in this issue. Management of autoimmune movement disorders consist of immunotherapy (dealt with in another section of this issue), removal of tumor whenever it is detected and feasible, and symptomatic treatment of the movement disorder manifestation. The symptomatic treatments which could be tried in movement disorders of autoimmune etiology are summarized in Table 2.

Parainfectious Autoimmune Movement Disorders

Sydenham's Chorea

Also known as rheumatic chorea, it is the most common cause of an acute or subacute onset isolated chorea in childhood. It is a prototype choreatic disorder with other classical accompaniments of chorea like motor impersistence (inability to maintain sustained muscle contraction) and hypotonia. The hypotonia is sometimes severe enough to hinder voluntary movement ("chorea paralytica"). Saccadic abnormalities, oculogyric crisis, and neuropsychiatric abnormalities like hyperactivity, obsessive compulsive disorder, and psychosis could occur in some cases. The chorea could be asymmetrical in around 20% of patients.

Sydenham's chorea (SC) occur as part of rheumatic fever (RF), which results from autoimmunity triggered by group A β-hemolytic streptococcal infection. Chorea is seen in

TABLE 2: Symptomatic treatments that can be tried for movement disorders of autoimmune etiology

Movement disorder	Symptomatic treatment
Parkinsonism	Levodopa, dopamine agonists (bromocriptine, pramipexole, ropinirole), and amantadine
Dystonia	Anticholinergics (trihexyphenidyl, benztropine), benzodiazepines, baclofen, tetrabenazine, levodopa, botulinum toxin injections
Tremor	Levodopa and dopamine agonists (Parkinsonian tremor and Holmes tremor), anticholinergics, botulinum toxin injections (dystonic tremor), propranolol, clonazepam, topiramate, isoniazid, and buspirone
Chorea	Tetrabenazine, typical antipsychotics (e.g., haloperidol, fluphenazine), atypical antipsychotics (e.g., risperidone, clozapine), benzodiazepines, amantadine, and anticonvulsants (like sodium valproate—particularly for rheumatic chorea)
Tics	Tetrabenazine, clonidine, antipsychotics (e.g., pimozide, risperidone), and benzodiazepines (clonazepam)
Myoclonus	Benzodiazepines, sodium valproate, piracetam, and levetiracetam

less than 25% of patients with RF. Rheumatic carditis occurs in around two-thirds to three-fourths of cases. No specific causative antibodies responsible for the CNS inflammation have been conclusively shown so far. MRI is normal in the majority but may show signal changes and swelling of basal ganglia structures in severe cases. SC may have a long-drawn course with remissions and relapses and accompanying neuropsychiatric morbidity. Symptomatic treatment to suppress chorea with antiepileptics (sodium valproate, carbamazepine) or neuroleptics like haloperidol is effective. Immunotherapy (steroids, plasma exchange, and intravenous immunoglobulin) is given in severe cases and may shorten the course and could lessen neuropsychiatric morbidity. Antibiotic prophylaxis for RF may be provided as per guidelines.

Acute or subacute onset of neuropsychiatric symptoms (emotional lability, irritability, anxiety, obsessive compulsive traits, etc.) accompanied sometimes by movement disorders (particularly, tics) occur in some children, precipitated by infections. Remissions and relapses occur. These were attributed to autoimmunity related to streptococcal infections and the term "PANDAS" (pediatric autoimmune neuropsychiatric disorder associated with streptococcal infections) was coined to describe the same. The specific link with streptococcal infection was challenged by many, and several other bacterial or viral infections were shown to be associated and hence, the terminology was later changed to pediatric acute-onset neuropsychiatric syndrome (PANS) or childhood acute neuropsychiatric syndrome (CANS). Treatment of the infection and symptomatic treatment are recommended and there are no clear guidelines on immunotherapy, for these entities.

Autoimmune Basal Ganglia Encephalitis

This is a relatively rare childhood autoimmune movement disorder. Contrary to the other conditions described above, Parkinsonism (akinesia and tremor) dominates the clinical picture in this condition, accompanied by hyperkinetic movement disorders like chorea and dystonia; sleep and neuropsychiatric disturbances, and dysautonomia are also usual accompaniments. This could follow a variety of infections like mycoplasma, group A streptococcus, influenza, and Epstein–Barr virus. Unlike similar clinical presentations by direct viral infection of basal ganglia structures (as in Japanese B encephalitis), autoimmune basal ganglia encephalitis shows presence of oligoclonal bands in cerebrospinal fluid (CSF), without any evidence for the infective agent as such, and responds to immunomodulation with steroids.

Paraneoplastic and Idiopathic Autoimmune Movement Disorders

Though the syndromes described below are associated with malignancy, they could also occur as idiopathic or postinfectious disorders.

Anti-N-methyl-D-aspartate Receptor Encephalitis

Anti-N-methyl-D-aspartate (NMDA) receptor encephalitis was initially described in young women as a paraneoplastic syndrome associated with ovarian teratoma. However, it was later recognized that this encephalitis syndrome could occur in children and older adults of both sexes though females are more commonly affected, and can occur as a paraneoplastic manifestation in response to malignancies involving organs like lungs, testes, pancreas, and the thymus gland as well. It can occur without tumors, particularly in children in whom the encephalitis can be idiopathic or infection-associated.

Anti-NMDA receptor encephalitis presents as a florid encephalitis syndrome with fever, neuropsychiatric, and autonomic manifestations, seizures and depressed level of alertness. Presentation with acute psychosis is not uncommon. The movement disorder of NMDA encephalitis is typically a mixture of hyperkinetic disorders, some of which may be difficult to classify into any of the classical hyperkinetic movement disorder phenomenologies listed in Table 1. Orofacial dyskinesia is a characteristic feature, often accompanied by choreodystonic and ballistic movements, and rhythmic or semi-rhythmic movements involving craniofacial musculature. The symptoms generally respond well to immunotherapy and removal of the tumor, if detected. Relapses could occur particularly in cases not associated with tumor and prolonged immunotherapy may be needed.

Opsoclonus-Myoclonus Syndrome

Opsoclonus-myoclonus syndrome (OMS) could occur in children as well as adults as a paraneoplastic, postinfectious or idiopathic disorder. Around 50% of cases in children are tumor associated and neuroblastoma is the commonest; the associated tumors in adults include small cell carcinoma of lung, breast cancer, and ovarian and testicular tumors. The hallmarks of the syndrome, as the name implies, are opsoclonus and myoclonus. Opsoclonus refers to involuntary saccadic eye movements which are totally chaotic and multidirectional. The myoclonus in OMS involves the facial, trunk, and limb musculature, and is exaggerated by action. Ataxia, encephalopathy, and behavioral changes are common accompaniments. In adults, lymphoma and leukemia could be associated with a similar syndrome with myoclonus, ataxia, and sleep disturbances; opsoclonus may not be a prominent feature. Response to immunotherapy and tumor removal is satisfactory.

Stiff Person Syndrome

This typically presents in middle ages and women are affected twice as commonly as men are. Rigidity of the proximal limb and trunk muscles with fluctuations in intensity and superadded spasms is the core clinical feature. Rigidity of paraspinal muscles result in exaggerated lumbar lordosis. The spasms are painful and are generally precipitated by auditory or tactile stimuli and emotional excitement.

Stiff person syndrome (SPS) could be a paraneoplastic syndrome associated with Hodgkin's lymphoma and cancers of lung, breast, and colon or idiopathic; co-occurrence with other autoimmune disorders like pernicious anemia, vitiligo, and autoimmune endocrinopathies including type 1 diabetes is well known. The onset of SPS is generally insidious and the course is chronic and progressive. Progressive encephalomyelitis with rigidity and myoclonus (PERM) is a more fulminant form with autonomic dysfunction and encephalopathy and evidence of more florid inflammation in CSF study and MRI. Rare pediatric cases of PERM have been reported. SPS and PERM require prolonged immunotherapy along with symptomatic medications including benzodiazepines and other GABAergic medications.

Paraneoplastic Chorea and Dystonia

Chorea is one among the manifestations of anti-collapsin response-mediated protein (CRMP)-5 encephalitis syndrome, which is paraneoplastic in majority of cases. Small cell cancer of the lung and thymic malignancies are the most common associations. The disorder could manifest as chorea alone or along with features of more extensive encephalon and peripheral involvement, like limbic encephalitis, cerebellar degeneration, and neuropathy. MRI is generally abnormal and the extent and distribution of hyperintensities vary parallel to variations in clinical presentation. Rare cases of cranio-cervical dystonia (jaw, neck, and larynx) have been described in women with breast cancer.

Paraneoplastic Parkinsonism

Parkinsonism is very rare as a paraneoplastic manifestation, but can occur in anti-Ma2 encephalitis. The common tumor associations are testicular germ cell tumors, cancers of breast and colon, lymphoma, and lung cancer of non-small cell type. The encephalon is affected diffusely. Therefore, Parkinsonism almost never occurs as an isolated phenomenon and is accompanied by memory disturbances and seizures (limbic region involvement), autonomic, sleep and hypothalamic dysfunction (resulting from diencephalon involvement), oculomotor dysfunction, other cranial neuropathies, and ataxia. The accompanying features and subacute onset help to differentiate it from the much more common, neurodegenerative forms of Parkinsonism. MRI is frequently abnormal. Immunotherapy is administered along with symptomatic treatment.

Movement Disorders Associated with Systemic Autoimmune Disorders

Among the systemic autoimmune disorders which could affect the CNS, antiphospholipid syndrome (APS) and systemic lupus erythematosus (SLE) can cause chorea, particularly in women. It is a relatively rare manifestation and can occur in only around 2–3% of patients. MRI is usually normal. Direct antibody-mediated neuronal injury is believed to be the mechanism of neurological dysfunction. The treatment consists of immunotherapy along with symptomatic treatment of chorea. There are also reports of rare cases of Parkinsonism and dystonia (particularly, blepharospasm, cervical dystonia) associated with SLE and improving with immunotherapy. Celiac disease (CD) or gluten sensitivity (GS) and Sjögren's syndrome (SS) are the other autoimmune disorders associated with movement disorders. CD and GS can cause ataxia, and SS is reported to cause Parkinsonism. Chorea and dystonia are the other movement disorders associated with SS.

DIAGNOSTIC APPROACH

Autoimmunity is a relatively uncommon etiology for movement disorders. Diagnosis may be easy when clinical presentations fit with a classical autoimmune movement disorder syndrome (like SC or anti-NMDA receptor encephalitis). In general, autoimmune etiology should be suspected when movement disorders have an acute or subacute presentation. Mixed movement disorders, movement disorders evolving subacutely along with clinical features of cerebellar, brainstem, limbic, or diencephalon involvement and those occurring in the background of a diagnosed malignancy are some of the clinical scenarios where autoimmunity should be investigated. Evidence of inflammation in CSF study or MRI also favors an autoimmune etiology. Targeted antibody testing or antibody panels should be ordered based on the clinical presentation. It should be remembered that the sensitivity of the autoantibody tests is not always absolute; empirical immunotherapy may therefore be justified in highly suggestive clinical settings even if autoantibody testing is negative, after discussing with the patient and family. An aggressive search for malignancy should be done when the clinical picture fits in with a paraneoplastic syndrome, particularly if autoantibody testing is positive. The autoantibody and tumor associations of autoimmune movement disorders are listed in Table 3. The autoantibodies could be onconeuronal

TABLE 3: Etiological factors and autoantibodies associated with autoimmune movement disorders

Clinical syndrome	Etiological factors	Autoantibody associations
Sydenham's chorea	Group A β-hemolytic streptococcal infection	Anti-basal ganglia, anti-tubulin, antiganglioside and dopamine receptor antibodies (role as a marker and in the pathogenesis of chorea is controversial). Serological evidence of streptococcal infection is usually present
PANS/ CANS	Bacterial/viral infections	Nil
Autoimmune basal ganglia encephalitis	Mycoplasma, influenza and Epstein–Barr virus infections, infections by group A streptococcus	Anti-dopamine D2 receptor
Anti-NMDAR encephalitis	Ovarian teratoma (young women); malignancies of lungs, testes, pancreas and the thymus gland; parainfectious; idiopathic	Antibodies against NR-1 subunit of NMDAR
Opsoclonus-myoclonus syndrome or paraneoplastic myoclonus	Neuroblastoma (children); parainfectious; idiopathic; small cell carcinoma of lung, cancers of breast, ovary and testes in adults; lymphoma	No autoantibody associations shown convincingly in children. Anti-Ri (ANNA-2-commonest) and anti-Ma1 and Ma2, anti-Hu and anti-DPPX in adults
Stiff person syndrome/ PERM	Paraneoplastic (Hodgkin's lymphoma and cancers of lung, breast and colon) or idiopathic; association with systemic autoimmune disorders	Anti-GAD65, anti-GlyR, anti-GABA-A receptor associated protein, anti-amphiphysin, and anti-DPPX
Paraneoplastic chorea	Small cell cancer of the lung; thymic malignancies, lymphoma	Anti-CRMP-5, anti-Hu (ANNA-1)
Paraneoplastic Parkinsonism	Testicular tumors, cancers of breast and colon, lymphoma, non-small cell lung cancer	Anti-Ma1 and Ma2
Movement disorders in systemic autoimmune diseases	SLE and APS, celiac disease / gluten sensitivity; Sjogren's syndrome	Antiphospholipid antibodies, antinuclear antibodies; anti-Gliadin, anti-Ro and anti-La; antibodies against neurofilaments, gangliosides and glial fibrillary acidic protein have been described in SLE but association with movement disorders not proven

NMDAR, N-methyl-D-aspartate receptor; CRMP-5, collapsin response-mediated protein-5; ANNA, anti-neuronal nuclear antibody; DPPX, dipeptidyl peptidase-like protein-6; GAD, glutamic acid decarboxylase; GlyR, glycine receptor; GABA, gamma-aminobutyric acid; PERM, progressive encephalomyelitis with rigidity and myoclonus; SLE, systemic lupus erythematosus; APS, antiphospholipid syndrome; CANS, childhood acute neuropsychiatric syndrome; PANS, pediatric acute-onset neuropsychiatric syndrome.

(directed against neuronal intracellular antigens; e.g., anti-CRMP-5) or targeting neuronal cell surface antigens (e.g., anti-NMDA R). The reader is referred to the relevant section of this issue for a discussion on different classes of antibodies and their pathogenic significance.

CONCLUSION

Identification of an autoimmune etiology, though not very common except for certain childhood syndromes like SC, is important as this forms a subgroup of potentially treatable or even curable movement disorders. The diagnosis is relatively easy when the patient presents with typical clinical syndromes. A high index of suspicion is needed for timely identification when the presentation does not fit fully with classical descriptions. Identification of the movement disorder phenomenology and associated other neurological manifestations help to arrive at a syndromic diagnosis which will guide further diagnostic work-up including autoantibody testing and search for tumor associations.

TAKE HOME MESSAGES

- Movement disorders are clinical manifestations resulting from dysfunction of circuits involving the basal ganglia structures and/or their connections
- Movement disorders can be classified phenomenologically into hypokinetic/bradykinetic disorders and hyperkinetic/dyskinetic disorders
- Autoimmune movement disorders are uncommon but constitute a subgroup of potentially treatable or even curable movement disorders
- They occur in pediatric as well as adult populations and can be paraneoplastic, parainfectious, idiopathic, or associated with other systemic autoimmune disorders
- Proper identification of the movement disorder phenomenology is important for making a syndromic diagnosis and planning investigations
- Presentation with any of the classical syndromes (described in text), acute or subacute onset, presence of mixed phenomenologies, changes suggestive of inflammation in CSF study and imaging, and background history of diagnosed malignancy or systemic autoimmune disorder should raise the suspicion of an underlying autoimmune etiology for the movement disorder
- Management consists of immunotherapy combined with symptomatic treatments aimed at relief of the movement disorder.

SUGGESTED READINGS

1. Abdo WF, van de Warrenburg BPC, Burn DJ, et al. The clinical approach to movement disorders. Nat Rev Neurol. 2010;6(1):29-37.
2. Baizabal-Carvallo JF, Jankovic J. Movement disorders in autoimmune diseases. Mov Disord Off J Mov Disord Soc. 2012;27(8):935-46.
3. Balint B, Vincent A, Meinck HM, et al. Movement disorders with neuronal antibodies: syndromic approach, genetic parallels and pathophysiology. Brain. 2018;141(1):13-36.
4. Cardoso F, Eduardo C, Silva AP, et al. Chorea in fifty consecutive patients with rheumatic fever. Mov Disord Off J Mov Disord Soc. 1997;12(5):701-3.
5. Dalmau J, Tüzün E, Wu H, et al. Paraneoplastic anti-N-methyl-D-aspartate receptor encephalitis associated with ovarian teratoma. Ann Neurol. 2007;61(1):25-36.
6. Giedd JN, Rapoport JL, Kruesi MJ, et al. Sydenham's chorea: magnetic resonance imaging of the basal ganglia. Neurology. 1995;45(12):2199-202.

7. Hero B, Schleiermacher G. Update on pediatric opsoclonus myoclonus syndrome. Neuropediatrics. 2013;44(6):324-9.
8. Honorat JA, McKeon A. Autoimmune Movement Disorders: a Clinical and Laboratory Approach. Curr Neurol Neurosci Rep. 2017;17(1):4.
9. Hutchinson M, Waters P, McHugh J, et al. Progressive encephalomyelitis, rigidity, and myoclonus: a novel glycine receptor antibody. Neurology. 2008;71(16):1291-2.
10. Lim TT. Paraneoplastic autoimmune movement disorders. Parkinsonism Relat Disord. 2017;44:106-9.
11. Luque FA, Furneaux HM, Ferziger R, et al. Anti-Ri: an antibody associated with paraneoplastic opsoclonus and breast cancer. Ann Neurol. 1991;29(3):241-51.
12. McKeon A, Robinson MT, McEvoy KM, et al. Stiff-man syndrome and variants: clinical course, treatments, and outcomes. Arch Neurol. 2012;69(2):230-8.
13. Mohammad SS, Fung VSC, Grattan-Smith P, et al. Movement disorders in children with anti-NMDAR encephalitis and other autoimmune encephalopathies. Mov Disord Off J Mov Disord Soc. 2014;29(12):1539-42.
14. Mohammad SS, Ramanathan S, Brilot F, et al. Autoantibody-associated movement disorders. Neuropediatrics. 2013;44(6):336-45.
15. Panzer J, Dalmau J. Movement disorders in paraneoplastic and autoimmune disease. Curr Opin Neurol. 2011;24(4):346-53.
16. Pittock SJ, Parisi JE, McKeon A, et al. Paraneoplastic jaw dystonia and laryngospasm with antineuronal nuclear autoantibody type 2 (anti-Ri). Arch Neurol. 2010;67(9):1109-15.
17. Postuma RB, Berg D, Stern M, et al. MDS clinical diagnostic criteria for Parkinson's disease. Mov Disord Off J Mov Disord Soc. 2015;30(12):1591-601.
18. Saiz A, Blanco Y, Sabater L, et al. Spectrum of neurological syndromes associated with glutamic acid decarboxylase antibodies: diagnostic clues for this association. Brain J Neurol. 2008;131(Pt 10):2553-63.
19. Samii A, Dahlen DD, Spence AM, et al. Paraneoplastic movement disorder in a patient with non-Hodgkin's lymphoma and CRMP-5 autoantibody. Mov Disord Off J Mov Disord Soc. 2003;18(12):1556-8.
20. Singer HS, Gilbert DL, Wolf DS, et al. Moving from PANDAS to CANS. J Pediatr. 2012;160(5):725-31.
21. Tan EK, Chan LL, Auchus AP. Reversible parkinsonism in systemic lupus erythematosus. J Neurol Sci. 2001;193(1):53-7.

CHAPTER 8

Autoimmune Cerebellar Ataxias

Sujin Koshy, Rajesh Shankar Iyer

INTRODUCTION

Autoimmune reactions of the central nervous system (CNS) can be diffuse as in multiple sclerosis or can target specific region(s), limbic system and cerebellum being two preferred targets. A clinical category of immune-mediated cerebellar ataxias (IMCAs) has been recognized recently in the last three decades.

HISTORICAL BACKGROUND

The role of immune-mediated pathogenesis in the etiology of cerebellar ataxia (CA) was first put forward by JM Charcot in the context of multiple sclerosis when he described the Charcot's triad (intention tremor, scanning speech, and nystagmus). In the last years, many have described cases with the cerebellum as the only target of autoimmunity, such as paraneoplastic cerebellar degeneration, the first cases of which were reported in 1919 by Brouwer and was secondary to ovarian carcinoma. The concept of nonparaneoplastic immune-mediated CAs was only established recently and was classified based on the antibody type [antibodies to glutamic acid decarboxylase (GAD), thyroid tissue, or gliadin]. Primary autoimmune cerebellar ataxia (PACA) has been recently introduced, where the cerebellum is a primary target of autoimmunity and may be associated with cerebellar autoantibodies.

PATHOGENESIS

The main pathological mechanism of Hashimoto's encephalopathy (HE) and ataxia in systemic lupus erythematosus is presumed to be vasculitis. The pathogenic agents are autoantibodies in anti-GAD antibody associated CA and Miller Fisher syndrome, and probably also in gluten ataxia. Cell-mediated autoimmunity is likely responsible for CAs in paraneoplastic cerebellar degeneration, autoantibodies are markers, but not the pathogenic agents. The specific mechanisms of the autoimmunity in each disease require further discussion.

CLASSIFICATION

Autoimmunity Targeting Mainly the Cerebellum or Related Structures

Cerebellar Autoimmunity Triggered by another Disease or Condition
- Gluten ataxia (gluten sensitivity)
- Acute cerebellitis (infection)
- Miller Fisher syndrome (infection)
- Paraneoplastic cerebellar degenerations (neoplasm).

Cerebellar Autoimmunity Not Triggered by another Disease or Condition
- Anti-GAD65 antibody-associated cerebellar ataxias
- Steroid-responsive IMCAs with antithyroid antibodies
- Primary autoimmune cerebellar ataxia
- Others.

Autoimmunity That Targets Various Parts of the Central Nervous System Simultaneously
- Multiple sclerosis
- Ataxia in the context of connective tissue diseases such as systemic lupus erythematosus.

Gluten Ataxia

It was earlier defined as idiopathic sporadic ataxia with circulating immunoglobulin (Ig) G or IgA antigliadin antibodies, but later antibodies more specific to neurological manifestations (anti-transglutaminase antibodies/anti-TG6 antibody) were identified. Presents usually as pure cerebellar ataxia but it can present with ataxia in combination with focal myoclonus, opsoclonus, or palatal tremor. Mean age at onset is 53 years and it usually has an insidious onset; however, can sometimes mimic paraneoplastic cerebellar degeneration with a rapidly progressive ataxia. Lower limb ataxia is common. Ocular signs including gaze evoked nystagmus are seen in about 80% of cases. A few having gastrointestinal symptoms like dyspepsia showed features of enteropathy on biopsy.

Cerebellar atrophy on magnetic resonance imaging (MRI) is seen in 60% of patients, but all patients have spectroscopic abnormalities affecting the vermis. Volumetric analysis of the cerebellum reveals significant abnormalities in those with celiac disease (CD) when compared to healthy controls.

Response to gluten-free diet depends on the duration of ataxia prior to the diagnosis. Loss of Purkinje cells due to prolonged gluten exposure is irreversible and early treatment is more likely to result in improvement of the ataxia.

Patients with myoclonic ataxia and CD often have enteropathy nonresponsive to the diet and are at risk of developing lymphoma. Both ataxia and enteropathy respond well to immunosuppressive treatment; however, myoclonus is poorly responsive and is the most disabling feature of this condition.

Acute Cerebellitis

Cerebellitis refers to an immune-mediated acute inflammation of the cerebellum. It is generally considered as postinfectious cerebellitis but it may at times mark the onset of PACA. Predominantly seen in children and is associated commonly with viral illnesses especially varicella. In adults, the commonest preceding infection is Epstein-Barr virus or mycoplasma. Acute cerebellitis is also seen after pertussis, typhoid, diphtheria, leptospirosis, mycoplasma, and Legionnaire's disease.

The clinical features include acute onset of cerebellar dysfunction, frequently associated with disorientation. Children can have severe ataxia resulting in inability to walk and the peak incidence is at 3 years. Full recovery can occur in 88% by 2 months. Adults can in addition have oculomotor disturbances and the latency from prodromal symptoms to ataxia was 3.5 weeks.

Cerebrospinal fluid examination shows elevation of white cell count (lymphocytes predominant), in 50% of patients and high protein in about 30% of patients. The MRI may demonstrate cerebellar swelling, atrophy is seen in those with incomplete recovery (18%). Incomplete recovery may indicate that acute cerebellitis is a primary autoimmune phenomenon leading to permanent and progressive ataxia, which is supported by the specificity in the involvement of cerebellum, sparing other parts of the brain.

The treatment should be started at the earliest targeting the etiologic agent. When the etiological agent is not clear or if complications are present (hydrocephalus and tonsillar herniation), mannitol, and steroids are indicated.

Cerebellar-like Ataxia in Miller Fisher Syndrome and Related Conditions

Richter in 1962, described the ataxic form of polyradiculoneuritis (Landry-Guillain-Barré syndrome), characterized by profound ataxia without weakness, no or minimal ophthalmoplegia, no sensory loss (especially of proprioception), and no Romberg sign. This clinical presentation is very similar to Miller Fisher syndrome except for the absence of ophthalmoplegia. The presence of anti-GQ1b IgG antibodies in ataxic Guillain-Barré syndrome as well as Miller Fisher syndrome identified that ataxic Guillain-Barré syndrome is an incomplete form of Miller Fisher syndrome.

The search for pathological involvement has identified the peripheral sensory nerve as one of the sites, the nature of damage is axonal and not demyelination. Some patients have striking limb in coordination with jerky rhythmical eye movements not influenced by eye closure, without any objective sensory changes, and a negative Romberg sign. Even though there is no nystagmus or cerebellar dysarthria, this form of ataxia seemed to be of cerebellar origin.

The MRI has shown enhancing lesions in the spinocerebellar tracts at the level of the lower medulla which also suggests that the cerebellar-like ataxia may be caused by selective involvement of group Ia afferents, from muscle spindles to spinal cord, or involvement of the spinocerebellar pathway.

Ataxia usually resolves within a few months, and near complete recovery can occur in 6 months. Immunomodulatory therapies (intravenous Ig and plasmapheresis) may hasten time to recovery and may decrease the likelihood of complications.

Paraneoplastic Cerebellar Degenerations

Paraneoplastic neurological syndromes (PNSs) represent remote effects of a cancer and they cannot be explained by metastatic, metabolic, iatrogenic, or infectious causes. Paraneoplastic cerebellar degenerations (PCDs) are the most frequently reported PNSs (24%).

Onset is usually subacute, with rare acute stroke-like presentations. Patients with PCDs present with symmetrically distributed static and kinetic cerebellar symptoms. Although isolated cerebellar ataxia is the most common presentation, extracerebellar (limbic regions, brainstem, spinal cord, or dorsal root ganglia) symptoms can occasionally be present. In 84% of the patients, the neurological syndrome precedes the discovery of the underlying tumor. Cerebrospinal fluid analysis may show mild lymphocytosis, increased proteins, and/or oligoclonal bands. The MRI is usually normal at the onset of disease, but during the later stages, cerebellar atrophy especially of the vermis can occur. Alternative diagnoses that should be excluded include cerebellar tumor, stroke, metabolic disease, leptomeningeal metastasis, late-onset degenerative cerebellar atrophy, infectious cerebellitis, and chemotherapy adverse effects.

Approximately 80% of the PCDs are associated with the onconeural antibodies (ONA), such as anti-Hu, anti-Yo, anti-CV2/collapsin response-mediator protein-5(CRMP5), anti-Ma2, anti-Ri, or anti-Tr delta/Notch-like epidermal growth factor-related receptor antibodies, emphasizing the role of autoimmune origin. Gynecologic malignancies (breast, ovaries, and uterus), small cell lung carcinoma and Hodgkin's lymphoma are the most frequent primary sites and each autoantibody associates with specific tumor types guiding in identification of the causative cancer.

The pathophysiological function of onconeuronal antibodies is still under debate. They may not play a role by themselves and probably act as a biological marker of the autoimmune process than having a direct role. The Purkinje cell death seen is supposed to be mainly due to a cell-mediated cytotoxic immune response. Brain biopsies have shown the presence of CD8+ T-cells infiltrates and activated microglia associated with a profound loss of Purkinje cells.

Neurological improvement is rare due to the diffuse neuronal loss and treatments allow only for a stabilization of the symptoms. Prognosis also varies depending on the nature of the associated ONA. Tumor removal and physiotherapy are the mainstay of treatment, immunotherapy is often ineffective. There may be subgroups of patients with anti-Hu or anti-Yo antibodies having a better response to immunotherapy, according to a few retrospective studies conducted.

Cerebellar Ataxia with Glutamic Acid Decarboxylase Autoantibodies

Glutamic acid decarboxylase is the rate-limiting enzyme for the production of γ-amino butyric acid (GABA), GAD is expressed in CNS GABAergic neurons and in the pancreatic islet β-cells and exists as two isoforms, GAD65 and GAD67. The GAD antibody is considered as the biological marker of type 1 diabetes mellitus (T1DM) and has also been reported in some neurological diseases including cerebellar ataxia.

This rare syndrome affects mostly females in their sixth decade, has an insidious or subacute onset, and tends to continuously progress over time. Symptoms include nystagmus, static ataxia, and dysarthria. The disorder may coexist with stiff person syndrome (SPS), peripheral neuropathy, limb stiffness, and myasthenia gravis and a personal or familial history of other autoimmune diseases (T1DM, hemolytic anemia, or thyroiditis) is frequent.

Brain MRI shows cerebellar atrophy, in those patients without SPS. Cerebrospinal fluid analysis may reveal oligoclonal bands and intrathecal synthesis of GAD antibodies. Usually the prognosis is poor with significant disability. More large-scale randomized studies are needed to determine the optimal therapeutic strategies. Immune therapy is the main stay of treatment. Intravenous immunoglobulins, if not corticosteroids, may have a beneficial effect in some patients, plasma exchange and immunosuppressive agents are the other options.

Cerebellar Type of Hashimoto's Encephalopathy

Approximately 28% of patients with HE may present with cerebellar ataxia. The age of onset ranged from 38 to 84 years, males being more commonly affected (8–10 times) and majority have an insidious onset; however, a stroke-like acute presentation is also seen.

Almost all the patients had truncal ataxia, but nystagmus appeared only in about 17% of patients. Those patients who presented with anti-NAE (NH2-terminal of α-enolase) antibodies tend to respond better to immune therapy than anti-NAE antibody negative patients.

Serum anti-TG and/or anti-thyroid peroxidase antibodies were detected in all patients, and serum anti-NAE antibodies were also detected in few. Most patients had elevated protein in cerebrospinal fluid, slow waves in electroencephalography are common; however, cerebral atrophy is a rare finding. Shows good response to steroid and is recognized as treatable ataxia, a few cases may require immunoglobulins or immunosuppressants.

Primary Autoimmune Cerebellar Ataxia

Cerebellum can be a primary organ specific autoimmune disease, in addition to specific cerebellar disease entities where autoimmunity is triggered by another disease. Human lymphocyte antigen (HLA) type DQ2 is significantly high in patients with idiopathic sporadic ataxia, when compared to the genetically characterized ataxias and general population. The presence of antibodies can be a useful diagnostic aid, though HLA DQ2 allele is present in up to 35% of healthy population. Evidence of autoimmune diseases in the patient or their first-degree relatives may be a helpful pointer. Characterization of the cerebellar antibodies will be the best diagnostic marker for PACA. Assessing the response to immunosuppression may help in its consolidation as a disease entity. Magnetic resonance spectroscopy assessing the vermis and hemispheres is also an important tool.

Patients develop ataxia in their early 50s which is slowly progressive in most of the cases. Absence of autonomic involvement and the slower progression helps in differentiating it from other ataxias. Almost all the patients have cerebellar atrophy on MRI, severity of which depends on disease duration. Treatment with steroids is recommended in the case of cerebellar edema and hydrocephalus. Neurosurgical intervention may be necessary to prevent brain herniation.

Ataxia Associated with Systemic Lupus Erythematosus

Immunological mechanisms affect different parts of the central and peripheral nervous system and is not specific to the cerebellum. Cerebellar involvement is rare

(2%). The acute ataxia can be primary, as part of the neuropsychiatric systemic lupus erythematosus (NPSLE) or secondary due to acute disseminated encephalomyelitis, drug-related inflammatory damage, vasculitis or atypical infections, later being common (two times). Females in reproductive age group are primarily involved. The clinical presentation varies depending on the pathogenic mechanism and part of cerebellum involved. Acute ataxia in lupus may be either a focal involvement (vaso-occlusion resulting in ischemia, infarction, hemorrhage or vasogenic edema); or a diffuse cerebellar involvement (antibodies like anti- anti-double stranded DNA, cross reacting to N-Methyl-D-aspartic acid receptors mediating cerebellar dysfunction). Focal involvement present with ipsilateral limb and ocular ataxia with cerebellar hemispheric signs, often with associated brainstem involvement. Diffuse involvement presents acute/subacute pan cerebellar symptoms of bilateral limb, gait, and ocular ataxia often without other neurologic findings.

Magnetic resonance imaging is the investigation of choice. Diffuse cerebellar atrophy and volume loss along with diffuse cerebral, corpus callosal, and hippocampal atrophy. Periventricular and subcortical white matter lesions are the most common MRI findings. In pediatric lupus patients, the volume loss is maximum in patients with NPSLE in the first 4 years of disease manifestation. Functional studies (positron emission tomography/single-photon emission computed tomography) reveal patchy areas of dysfunction in brain areas unaffected in conventional MRI. Symptomatic therapy, anticoagulants, and immunosuppressive treatments are the mainstay of therapy. Antithrombotic therapy or control of hypertension may be needed for the stroke episodes, other cases of cerebellar ataxia require immunologic modification (steroids/cyclophosphamide) therapy. High-dose intravenous methyl prednisolone therapy is often effective, leading to the reversal of MRI abnormality before the clinical improvement.

CONCLUSION

Autoimmune cerebellar ataxias are triggered by unknown antigenic stimulants and strong suspicion is required for early diagnosis of the disease by the clinicians. Immune modulatory therapy is the main stay of treatment. However, the treatment response may vary according to etiology.

TAKE HOME MESSAGES

- Autoimmune cerebellar ataxias can be either paraneoplastic or nonparaneoplastic
- Gluten ataxia presents usually as pure cerebellar ataxia but it can present with ataxia in combination with focal myoclonus, opsoclonus, or palatal tremor
- Paraneoplastic cerebellar degenerations are the most frequently reported paraneoplastic syndromes and 80% of them are associated with ONAs
- Cerebellar ataxia with glutamic acid decarboxylase autoantibodies affects mostly females in their sixth decade and presents with nystagmus, static ataxia, and dysarthria
- Similar to hypothyroidism, primary autoimmune cerebellar ataxia is an organ specific autoimmune disease affecting the cerebellum
- Though immune modulatory therapy is the main stay of treatment, the treatment response is not uniform and vary according to etiology.

SUGGESTED READINGS

1. Ariño H, Gresa-Arribas N, Blanco Y, et al. Cerebellar ataxia and glutamic acid decarboxylase antibodies: Immunologic profile and long term effect of immunotherapy. JAMA Neurol. 2014;71:1009-16.
2. Bashir H, Ranganathan P. An unusual case of cerebellar haemorrhage inpatient with systemic lupus erythematosus. Arthritis Care Res (Hoboken). 2010;62:738-42.
3. Briani C, Vitaliani R, Grisold W, et al. Spectrum of paraneoplastic disease associated with lymphoma. Neurology. 2011;76:705-10.
4. Brouwer B. Beitrag zur kenntnis der chronischen diffusen kleinhirnerkranghkungen. Cent F¨ur Nervenheilkd Psychiatr Gerichtl Psychopathol. 1919;38:674-82.
5. Burk K, Melms A, Schulz JB, et al. Effectiveness of intravenous immunoglobulin therapy in cerebellar ataxia associated with gluten sensitivity. Ann Neurol. 2001;50:82
6. Charcot JM. Séancedu 14 mars. Cr Soc Biol (Paris).1868;20:13.
7. Chiba A, Kunosaki S, Shimizu T, et al. Serum IgG antibody to ganglioside GQ1b is a possible marker of Miller Fisher syndrome. Ann Neurol. 1992;31:677-9.
8. Chiba A, Kusunoki S, Obata H, et al. Serum anti-GQ1b IgG antibody is associated with ophthalmoplegia in Miller Fisher syndrome and Guillain-Barré syndrome: Clinical and immune histochemical studies. Neurology. 1993;43:1911-7.
9. Connolly AM, Dodson WE, Prensky AL, et al. Course and outcome of acute cerebellar ataxia. Ann Neurol. 1994;35:673-9.
10. Currie S, Hadjivassiliou M, Clark MJ, et al. Should we be 'nervous' about coeliac disease? Brain abnormalities in patients with coeliac disease referred for neurological opinion. J Neurol Neurosurg Psychiatry. 2012;83:1216-21.
11. Darnell RB, Posner JB. Paraneoplastic syndromes involving the nervous system. N Engl J Med. 2003;349:1543-54.
12. De Bruecker Y, Claus F, Demaerel P, et al. MRI findings in acute cerebellitis. Eur Radiol. 2004;14: 1478-83.
13. Diaconu G, Burlea M, Grigore I, et al.Celiac disease with neurologic manifestations in children. Rev Med Chir Med Nat Iasi. 2013;117:88-94.
14. Ducray F, Demarquay G, Graus F, et al. Seronegative paraneoplastic cerebellar degeneration: The PNS Euro network experience. Eur J Neurol. 2014;21:731-5.
15. Fisher M. An unusual variant of acute idiopathic polyneuritis (syndrome of ophthalmoplegia, ataxia and areflexia). N Engl J Med. 1956;255:57-65.
16. Giometto B, Grisold W, Vitaliani R, et al. Paraneoplastic neurologic syndrome in the PNS Euro network database: A European study from 20 centers. Arch Neurol. 2010;67:330-5.
17. Greenlee JE, Clawson SA, Hill KE, et al. Purkinje cell death after uptake of anti-Yo antibodies in cerebellar slice cultures. J Neuropathol Exp Neurol. 2010;69:997-1007.
18. Göhlich-Ratmann G, Wallot M, Baethmann M, et al. Acute cerebellitis with near-fatal cerebellar swelling and benign outcome under conservative treatment with high dose steroids. Eur J Paediatr Neurol. 1998;2(3):157-62.
19. Hadjivassiliou M, Aeschlimann P, Strigun A. Autoantibodies in gluten ataxia recognize a novel neuronal transglutaminase. Ann Neurol. 2008;64:332-43.
20. Hadjivassiliou M, Boscolo S, Davies Jones GA, et al. The humoral response in the pathogenesis of gluten ataxia. Neurology. 2002;58:1221-6.
21. Hadjivassiliou M, Boscolo S, Tongiorgi E, et al. Cerebellar ataxia as a possible organ specific autoimmune disease. Mov Disord. 2008;23:1270-377.
22. Hadjivassiliou M, Currie S, Hoggard N. MR spectroscopy in paraneoplastic cerebellar degeneration. J Neuroradiol. 2013;40: 310-2.
23. Honnorat J, Saiz A, Giometto B, et al. Cerebellar ataxia with anti-glutamic acid decarboxylase antibodies. Study of 14 patients. Arch Neurol. 2001;58:225-30.
24. Kheder A, Currie S, Romanowski C, et al. Progressive ataxia with palatal tremor due to gluten sensitivity. Mov Disord. 2012;27:62-3.
25. Klockgether T, Döller G, Wüllner U, et al. Cerebellar encephalitis in adults. J Neurol. 1993;240:17-20.
26. Manto M, Goldman S, Bodur H. Cerebellar syndrome associated with Hashimoto's encephalopathy. Rev Neurol (Paris). 1996;152: 202-4.

27. Matsunaga A, Ikawa M, Fujii A, et al. Hashimoto's encephalopathy as a treatable adult onset cerebellar ataxia mimicking spinocerebellar degeneration. Eur Neurol. 2013;69:14-20.
28. Mitoma H, Adhikari K, Aeschlimann D, et al. Consensus paper: Neuroimmune mechanisms of cerebellar ataxias. Cerebellum. 2016;15(2):213-32.
29. Muscal E, Traipe E, de Guzman MM, et al. Cerebral and cerebellar volume loss in children and adolescents with systemic lupus erythematosus: A review of clinically acquired brain magnetic resonance imaging. J Rheumatol. 2010;37:1768-75.
30. Nakagawa H, Yoneda M, Fujii A, et al. Hashimoto's encephalopathy presenting with progressive cerebellar ataxia. J Neurol Neurosurg Psychiatry. 2007;78:196-7.
31. Rakocevic G, Raju R, Semino-Mora C, et al. Stiff person syndrome with cerebellar disease and high-titer anti-GAD antibodies. Neurology. 2006;67:1068-70.
32. Richter RB. The ataxic form of polyradiculoneuritis (Landry Guillain-Barré syndrome). Clinical and pathologic observations. J Neuropathol Exp Neurol. 1962;21:171-84.
33. Saiz A, Arpa J, Sagasta A, et al. Autoantibodies to glutamic acid decarboxylase in three patients with cerebellar ataxia, late-onset insulin-dependent diabetes mellitus, and polyendocrine autoimmunity. Neurology. 1997;49:1026-30.
34. Selim M, Drachman DA. Ataxia associated with Hashimoto's disease: Progressive non-familial adult onset cerebellar degeneration with autoimmune thyroiditis. J Neurol Neurosurg Psychiatry. 2001;71:81-7.
35. Shams'ili S, Grefkens J, de Leeuw B, et al. Paraneoplastic cerebellar degeneration associated with antineuronal antibodies: analysis of 50 patients. Brain. 2003;126:1409-18.
36. Sibbitt WL, Brooks WL, Kornfeld M, et al. Magnetic brain imaging and brain histopathology in neuropsychiatric systemic lupus erythematosus. Semin Arthritis Rheum. 2010;40:32-52.
37. Storstein A, Krossnes BK, Vedeler CA. Morphological and immunohistochemical characterization of paraneoplastic cerebellar degeneration associated with Yo antibodies. Acta Neurol Scand. 2009;120:64-7.
38. Teh LS. Neuropsychiatric systemic lupus erythematosus (NPSLE). CPD Rheumatol. 2003;3:77-81.
39. Umapathi T, Tan EY, Kokubun N, et al. Non-demyelinating, reversible conduction failure in Fisher syndrome and related disorders. J Neurol Neurosurg Psychiatry. 2012;83:941-8.
40. Urushitani M, Udaka F, Kameyama M. Miller Fisher-Guillain Barré overlap syndrome with enhancing lesions in the spinocerebellar tracts. J Neurol Neurosurg Psychiatry. 1995;58: 241-3.
41. Yamamoto M, Wada-Isoe K, Yoneda M, et al. A case of acute cerebellar ataxia associated with serum anti-NH2 terminal of alpha-enolase (NAE) antibody. Rinsho Shinkeigaku. 2010;50:581-4.
42. Yoneda M, Fujii A, Ito A, et al. High prevalence of serum autoantibodies against the amino terminal of α-enolase in Hashimoto's encephalopathy. J Neuroimmunol. 2007;185:195-200.
43. Zuliani L, Sabater L, Saiz A, et al. Homer 3 autoimmunity in subacute idiopathic cerebellar ataxia. Neurology. 2007;68:239-40.

CHAPTER 9

Autoimmune Myelopathies

Mini Sreedharan, Kalpana D

INTRODUCTION

Autoimmune myelopathies constitute a heterogeneous group of disorders characterized by immune-mediated or immune-related injury to spinal cord. These include primary autoimmune myelopathies [neuromyelitis optica (NMO) or neuromyelitis optica spectrum disorders (NMOSD)], postinfectious or post vaccinial myelitis, paraneoplastic myelopathies, myelopathies associated with systemic autoimmune diseases and immune-related myelopathies [multiple sclerosis (MS), neurosarcoidosis, etc.]. Some of the autoimmune myelopathies like NMOSD, MS, paraneoplastic myelopathies, etc. have well-established diagnostic criteria.

Clinically, autoimmune myelopathies have many common symptoms and signs and these may be indistinguishable from those of nonimmune myelopathies. However, accompanying other systemic manifestations, magnetic resonance imaging (MRI) features, presence of autoantibodies, and the course are often helpful in narrowing down the differential diagnosis.

GENERAL FEATURES OF MYELOPATHY

Symptoms of myelopathy depend upon the segment of spinal cord affected and the longitudinal and transverse extent of lesions. The symptoms may evolve acutely or subacutely as in postinfectious myelitis, postvaccinial myelitis, NMOSD, myelitis with acute disseminated encephalomyelitis (ADEM), etc. or more slowly as in paraneoplastic myelopathy, primary progressive multiple sclerosis (PPMS), etc. The course may be monophasic (ADEM, post vaccinial myelitis), relapsing and remitting [NMOSD, relapsing-remitting multiple sclerosis (RRMS)] or chronic course (PPMS, paraneoplastic myelopathy).

In general, weakness and descending numbness (occasionally ascending) with a definite level (band-like sensation) are suggestive of spinal cord pathology. During initial stage of hyperacute myelitis, flaccid paralysis mimicking Guillain-Barré syndrome, numbness and absent reflexes, and mute plantar response are seen. Persistent urinary bladder retention and sensory levels often are pointers to spinal cord involvement. Later, the classical picture of lower motor neuron weakness (corresponding to segments at the upper level of lesion) and upper motor neuron weakness characterized by spasticity, exaggerated deep tendon reflexes and extensor plantar responses evolves. Increased pyramidal weakness on neck flexion (McArdle's sign) has been reported with cervical cord lesions. Autonomic disturbances including erectile dysfunction in males may also occur. Cervical cord involvement may result in respiratory muscle weakness and loss of facial pain sensation due to lesions affecting the descending tract and nucleus of trigeminal nerve. With NMO/NMOSD, the myelitis tends to be rather complete with bilateral severe deficits unlike MS with partial myelitis (Brown-Sequard syndrome).

Lhermitte's symptom (shock-like sensation shooting down the spine on neck flexion), heat-induced worsening of symptoms (Uhthoff's phenomenon), sensory useless hand (proprioceptive difficulty in using upper limb due to posterior tract involvement) are features suggestive of MS. Carbamazepine responsive paroxysmal tonic painful spasms characterized by recurrent painful dystonias especially of flexor muscles are more common with NMO/NMOSD than MS.

INDIVIDUAL AUTOIMMUNE MYELOPATHIES: CLINICAL FEATURES, COURSE AND INVESTIGATIONS

Neuromyelitis Optica or Neuromyelitis Optica Spectrum Disorders

Neuromyelitis optica is a well-defined clinical entity characterized by acute attacks of longitudinally extensive transverse myelitis (LETM) and optic neuritis. It was earlier known as Devic's disease or Asian opticospinal myelitis. Traditionally, it was thought to have a monophasic disease with concurrent or sequential occurrence of bilateral optic neuritis and transverse myelitis; but now it is well known that it has a wider spectrum of clinical manifestations and is termed NMOSD. Approximately 70–90% of NMOSD patients with LETM and optic neuritisa, and nearly half the patients with limited forms of NMOSD are positive for the pathogenic immunoglobulin G (IgG) autoantibody against aquaporin-4 (AQP4). Aquaporin-4 is a membrane protein which acts as water channel in central nervous system (CNS) and lesions of NMOSD tend to involve regions rich in AQP4. Aquaporin-4 antibody is highly specific for NMOSD and is a pathogenic antibody. The primary triggering immune event is unknown. The AQP4-IgG enters CNS through endothelial transcytosis or through breaks in blood brain barrier and binds to AQP4. This leads to downregulation of AQP4 and perturbed water homeostasis in the CNS. It also activates complement produced locally by astrocytes, which in turn leads to increased blood-brain barrier permeability and massive infiltration of leukocytes, particularly eosinophils and neutrophils. The combination of complement-mediated injury and cellular influx leads to the death of astrocytes, oligodendrocytes ,and neurons. The complement membrane attack complex also causes changes in local blood vessels including their irregular thickening and hyalinization. The role of myelin oligodendrocyte glycoprotein (MOG) antibody in pathogenesis is unclear. Clonal proliferation of B-cell is unusual and this explains the rare occurrence of elevated IgG in cerebrospinal fluid (CSF) in NMOSD.

Like the other autoimmune disorders, NMO is more common in females (4:1 to 9:1) in most series. The median age at onset is 30–40 years but older adults and children may also be affected. Unlike MS, non white ethnic group (African descent, Hispanics, Asians and Native Americans) are more susceptible.

Typically, NMO presents with either severe attacks of longitudinally extensive (≥3 vertebral segments) myelitis or optic neuritis (unilateral/bilateral) or both (4%). Older patients tend to present with myelitis while younger ones present with optic neuritis. The course is relapsing and remitting in majority and produces severe disability especially if seropositive for AQP4 antibody. Residual deficits result from recurrent attacks of myelitis and are not usually due a progressive course as seen in patients with MS. Neuromyelitis optica with monophasic course tends to be less severe and less frequent in females and is more common among younger age.

Box 1 shows the current International Panel for Neuromyelitis Optica Diagnostic Criteria for NMOSD. As per this, for patients with AQP4-IgG seropositivity, a single clinical

---

Box 1: International Panel for Neuromyelitis Optica (IPND) diagnostic criteria for NMO or NMOSD (2015)

Diagnostic criteria for NMOSD with AQP4-IgG
- At least one core clinical characteristic
- Positive test for AQP4-IgG using best available detection method (cell-based assay strongly recommended over immunofluorescence or ELISA)
- Exclusion of alternative diagnoses

Diagnostic criteria for NMOSD without AQP4-IgG or NMOSD with unknown AQP4-IgG status
- At least two core clinical characteristics occurring as a result of one or more clinical attacks and meeting all of the following requirements:
  - At least one core clinical characteristic must be optic neuritis, acute myelitis with LETM, or area postrema syndrome
  - Dissemination in space (more than or equal to two different core clinical characteristics)
  - Fulfillment of additional MRI requirements, as applicable
- Negative test(s) for AQP4-IgG using best available detection method, or testing unavailable
- Exclusion of alternative diagnoses

Core clinical characteristics
- Optic neuritis
- Acute myelitis
- Area postrema syndrome: Episode of otherwise unexplained hiccups or nausea and vomiting
- Acute brain stem syndrome
- Symptomatic narcolepsy or acute diencephalic clinical syndrome with NMOSD typical diencephalic MRI lesions
- Symptomatic cerebral syndrome with NMOSD-typical brain lesions

Additional MRI requirements for NMOSD without AQP4-IgG and NMOSD with unknown AQP4-IgG status
- Acute optic neuritis—requires brain MRI showing (a) normal findings or only nonspecific white matter lesions or (b) optic nerve MRI with T2-hyperintense lesion or T1-weighted gadolinium-enhancing lesion extending over more than half optic nerve length or involving optic chiasm
- Acute myelitis—requires associated intramedullary MRI lesion extending over three contiguous segments (LETM) or three contiguous segments of focal spinal cord atrophy in patients with prior history compatible with acute myelitis
- Area postrema syndrome—requires associated dorsal medulla/area postrema lesions
- Acute brain stem syndrome—requires associated periependymal brain stem Lesions

NMO, neuromyelitis optica; NMOSD, neuromyelitis optica spectrum disorders; ELISA, enzyme-linked immunosorbent assay; LETM, longitudinally extensive transverse myelitis; AQP4, aquaporin-4; IgG, immunoglobulin G ; MRI, magnetic resonance imaging.

event involving any one of six CNS regions (optic nerve, spinal cord, area postrema, brain stem, diencephalon, or cerebrum) is sufficient for diagnosis, when no alternative diagnosis can be offered. "Area postrema syndrome" manifesting as intractable nausea, vomiting, and/or hiccups due to a lesion in the dorsal medulla can occur in up to 40% of patients during the course of illness. Other manifestations of brain stem involvement can be ophthalmoplegia, hearing loss and opsoclonus/myoclonus. Symptoms due to "diencephalic involvement" include narcolepsy, syndrome of inappropriate antidiuretic hormone and eating disorders, temperature dysregulation and sham rage. Carbamazepine responsive tonic spasms, neurogenic pain or pruritus can occur. Encephalopathy and posterior reversible encephalopathy syndrome are also reported.

Myelin Oligodendrocyte Glycoprotein Positive Neuromyelitis Optica Spectrum Disorders

Nearly half of NMOSD patients seronegative for AQP4 have antibodies against MOG IgG. Its pathogenic role is not yet established and may be seen in some other autoimmune disorders like ADEM. Myelin oligodendrocyte glycoprotein-positive NMOSD patients tend to be younger, have simultaneous occurrence of bilateral optic neuritis and myelitis and respond well to immunotherapy. Myelitis affects lower cord segments (thoracolumbar) especially conus medullaris. The course is benign with lower relapse rate, a longer interval between subsequent attacks, and better functional recovery. There is no striking gender predilection.

Lesions of NMOSD are distributed in regions where AQP4 is highly expressed as evidenced by MRI. The MRI spine helps to differentiate various immune myelopathies. Longitudinally extensive transverse myelitis with T2-hyperintense lesion extending more than or equal to three vertebral segments on sagittal images is a hallmark feature of NMO. In AQP4 seropositive group, the lesions tend to be more in cervicothoracic region unlike in MOG-positive NMOSD where they involve lower cord. The lesions are usually central within the cord on axial images in contrast to MS lesions. Spinal cord swelling is common, and may be mistaken for tumor in some cases. Shorter lesions extending for fewer than three vertebral segments may occur infrequently, particularly in seronegative NMOSD or when imaging is done too early or too late. Other features, but not specific for NMOSD, include T1-hypointensity, extension of lesions towards the obex, and patchy gadolinium enhancement. Lesions may resolve completely, leave residual T2-signal abnormality, or result in focal or occasionally longitudinal extensive atrophy.

The MRI brain is abnormal in nearly 60% patients with NMOSD. The lesions include unilateral or bilateral T2-signal changes and gadolinium enhancement of the optic nerves which usually extend for more than or equal to half its length which may extend back to involve the optic chiasm, T2-signal abnormality with or without gadolinium enhancement in the region of area postrema and periependymal signal abnormalities surrounding the third and fourth ventricles. "Cloud-like" enhancement, posterior reversible encephalopathy-like lesions, extensive brain lesions mimicking ADEM and longitudinally extensive corpus callosum lesions different from the focal "Dawson finger" lesions typical of MS lesions are also reported in NMO. However, brain stem and supratentorial white matter lesions indistinguishable from those seen in MS are also seen in some patients.

Cerebrospinal fluid shows mild elevation in white blood cell (WBC) count in two-third cases of NMOSD. The cell types include lymphocytes, neutrophils, or eosinophils, which are also elevated in parasitic infections; CSF protein is typically elevated. Oligoclonal bands (OCB) or elevated IgG index are seen in less than 20% of NMOSD cases.

Postinfectious and Postimmunization Myelopathies

Acute disseminated encephalomyelitis is a monophasic inflammatory disease affecting the multiple sites in CNS, which usually follows an infection or vaccination. It is more common in children and young adults. The usual manifestations include encephalitis, seizures, cranial nerve palsies, meningeal signs, ataxia, hemiparesis, quadriparesis or paraparesis. Restricted forms of disease presenting as isolated transverse myelitis can occur. The MRI spine reveals either short segment or long segment lesions or may even be normal. Brain MRI often shows large and often confluent areas of cerebral or cerebellar white matter and deep gray (basal ganglia, thalamus) hyperintensity in T2 and fluid-attenuated inversion recovery (FLAIR) sequences (Fig. 1). Peripheral gadolinium enhancement may be seen. The CSF shows pleocytosis and transient elevation of OCB. Presence of myelitis in ADEM is reported to be a bad prognostic indicator for morbidity.

Paraneoplastic Myelopathies

This is a rare entity. The most common cancers associated with paraneoplastic isolated myelopathies are small-cell lung cancer and breast cancer. Autoantibodies are found in 81% of patients with paraneoplastic isolated myelopathy. Amphiphysin and

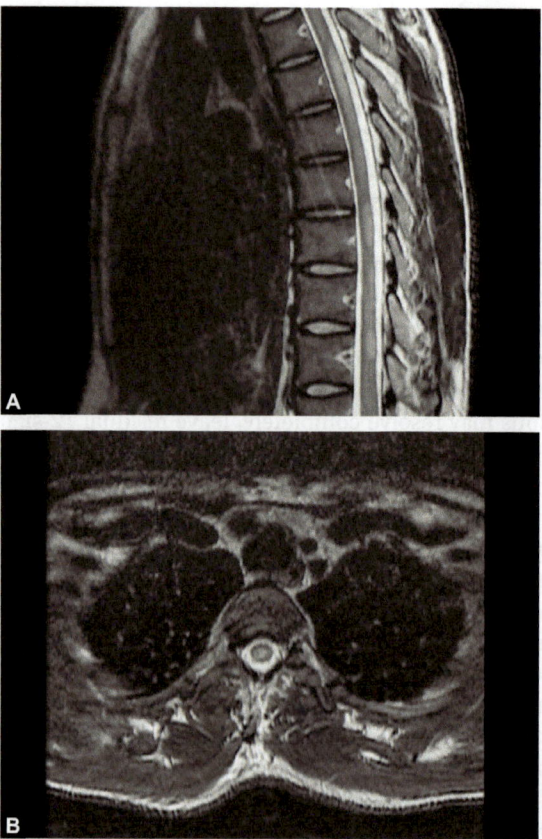

FIG. 1: A, T2 sequence showing longitudinally extensive transverse myelitis involving thoracic cord; **B,** Transverse section showing central hyperintensity.

collapsin response-mediator protein type-5-immunoglobulin G is the most common autoantibody associations, others include antineuronal nuclear antibodies-1 (ANNA-1) (anti-Hu), ANNA-2 (anti-Ri), ANNA-3 (anti-Yo), Purkinje cell antibody, anti-Ma, and anti-Ta. Weak association is reported with AQP4 antibody, voltage-gated potassium channel, etc. Symptoms are usually subacute in onset and may precede or follow the malignancy. It is common in elderly and course is progressive. The CSF shows pleocytosis and elevated protein and OCB. Nearly half of the patients show LETM. Tract specific contrast enhancement of the dorsal or lateral columns seen in nearly one-third patients is a hallmark feature of paraneoplastic myelopathy. It is usually associated with poor outcome.

Myelitis due to Multiple Sclerosis

Myelitis due to MS initially has a relapsing and remitting course and later develops a progressive course [secondary progressive multiple sclerosis (SPMS)]. However, some patients develop a progressive course after the initial attack (single attack progressive MS) or just present as a chronic, progressive myelopathy (PPMS). Readers may refer to chapter titled 'Autoimmune Demyelination' for detailed diagnostic criteria of MS.

The myelitis in RRMS is acute and partial and involves short segments (<3), usually along the periphery of the cord. Longitudinally extensive transverse myelitis is extremely rare in adults with MS but nearly 14% of pediatric MS patients show LETM. On the other hand, 14% patients with NMOSD may develop short segment myelitis even when timing of image is optimal. Brain MRI shows lesions suggestive of MS. Primary progressive multiple sclerosis affects elderly and is more frequent in males. They present with gradually progressive spastic paraparesis with no definite sensory levels. Patients with PPMS have fewer brain lesions compared to RRMS or SPMS. Cord atrophy occurs in PPMS, but is unusual in RRMS or SPMS. Gadolinium enhancement of lesions is infrequent in PPMS unlike RRMS. The CSF shows increased OCB or IgG index (Box 2).

Myelopathy in Sarcoidosis

About 10% patients with sarcoidosis present with neurological symptoms. Myelopathy due to sarcoidosis is often underdiagnosed. It causes LETM in nearly 77% cases. The MRI findings in T2 and FLAIR sequences are similar to NMOSD and other LETM. Intense homogeneous subpial enhancement in gadolinium sequences is a useful clue for sarcoid

---

Box 2: McDonald criteria for primary progressive multiple sclerosis (2010)

- One year of disease progression (retrospectively or prospectively determined)
- Plus two of the three following criteria:[a]
    - Evidence for DIS in the brain based on one T2b lesion in at least one area characteristic for MS (periventricular, juxta cortical, or infratentorial)
    - Evidence for DIS in the spinal cord based on two T2[b] lesions in the cord
    - Positive CSF (isoelectric focusing evidence of oligoclonal bands and/or elevated IgG index)

a–If a subject has a brainstem or spinal cord syndrome, all symptomatic lesions are excluded from the criteria.
b–Gadolinium enhancement of lesions is not required.

DIS, dissemination in space; MS, multiple sclerosis; CSF, cerebrospinal fluid.

myelopathy. The CSF often shows elevated WBC count and low CSF glucose levels. Elevated CSF angiotensin converting enzyme levels is seen only in minority of cases.

Autoimmune Myelopathies with Other Autoimmune Disorders

Autoimmune myelopathies have been described with a number of systemic autoimmune disorders like systemic lupus erythematosus, Sjogren's syndrome, Behcet's disease, scleroderma, anti-phospholipid antibody syndrome, etc. They may present as acute transverse myelitis or chronic myelopathy with longitudinally extensive spinal lesions in MRI. Accompanying systemic symptoms and signs and laboratory tests often give clue regarding the underlying systemic autoimmune disease.

There are reports that AQP4-positive NMOSD may develop in some patients with myasthenia gravis. Similarly, patients with N-Methyl-D-aspartate receptor encephalitis may develop NMOSD and vice versa.

DIFFERENTIAL DIAGNOSIS

Infectious myelitis, spondylotic myelopathy, vascular causes of myelopathy like ischemic neuritis and dural arteriovenous fistula, and intramedullary tumors, all can have similar clinical presentation. Careful examination, identifying MRI pattern and serological tests often help in confirming diagnosis.

TREATMENT

Early recognition of underlying autoimmune nature and targeted therapy is important for reducing morbidity and improving outcome. Initial therapy in NMOSD and RRMS include intravenous methyl prednisolone, intravenous immunoglobulin or plasma exchange, or rituximab. Maintenance therapy with high dose oral corticosteroids (1 mg/kg) along with steroid-sparing agent (azathioprine, mycophenolate mofetil, methotrexate, etc.) immediately after an attack helps in preventing recurrences. Distinguishing NMOSD from MS is very crucial for prognostication and therapy as the disease modifying drugs used for MS can actually worsen NMOSD (Table 1). Novel therapeutic agents for NMO under trial include interleukin-6 inhibitors like tocilizumab and complement inhibitors like eculizumab. For RRMS, conventional immunomodulatory therapies, such as interferon-beta and glatiramer acetate are used. For PPMS, drugs used include mitoxantrone,

TABLE 1: Features of neuromyelitis optica spectrum disorder versus multiple sclerosis

Feature	NMOSD	Multiple sclerosis
Ethnicity	Non-Caucasian	Caucasian
Carbamazepine responsive tonic spasms	Frequent	Rare
Pattern of myelitis	Longitudinally extensive (≥3 segments), lesions may extend to obex, lesions hyperintense in T2 and FLAIR, T1 hypointensity ±, patchy contrast enhancement, initial cord swelling and later atrophy	Usually short segment lesion (<3)

Continued

Continued

Feature	NMOSD	Multiple sclerosis
Transverse extent of spinal lesion	Central	Peripheral
MRI optic nerve	Involves more than half length of optic nerve, extends backwards involving chiasma	Shorter lesion, involves anterior part
Brain MRI lesions	Normal or typical lesions, along the distribution of AQP4, in the periependymal regions surrounding the third ventricle, cerebral aqueduct and fourth ventricle, thalamus, diencephalon, linear medullary lesions, cloud like cerebral lesions with patchy enhancement and blurred margins	Juxtacortical, periventricular lesions, perpendicular to corpus callosum
Serum AQP4-IgG	Positive in 70–90%	Absent
CSF OCB	Less frequent	Elevated

CSF, Cerebrospinal fluid; OCB, oligoclonal bands; AQP4, aquaporin-4; MRI, magnetic resonance imaging; FLAIR, fluid-attenuated inversion recovery; NMOSD, neuromyelitis optica spectrum disorder.

cladribine, methotrexate, etc. Treatment of underlying malignancy may produce some improvement in paraneoplastic myelopathy; however, overall prognosis is poor. Readers may refer to chapter titled 'Immunotherapy' for further details.

CONCLUSION

Autoimmune myelopathies are a diverse group of disorders with an immunological basis for the spinal cord pathology. Recognizing the specific MRI patterns and detection of associated autoantibodies and accompanying systemic manifestations help in better diagnosis and management.

TAKE HOME MESSAGES

- Autoimmune myelopathies form a heterogeneous group of disorders with immune mediated injury to spinal cord
- Recognizing the pattern of cord involvement by MRI (LETM vs. short segment transverse myelitis) is useful in differentiating various autoimmune myelopathies
- Longitudinally extensive central cord lesions are suggestive of NMOSD while short segment, peripheral lesions favor MS
- Tract specific hyperintensity would indicate paraneoplastic or nutritional myelopathy
- Serum AQP4-IgG antibody is highly specific for NMOSD
- Neuromyelitis optica spectrum disorder can present with wider spectrum of manifestations like area postrema syndrome, narcolepsy, etc.
- Differentiating between NMOSD and MS is imperative as immunomodulatory therapy used for MS may worsen NMOSD
- Nonimmune myelopathies may have similar clinical presentation and hence should be considered in differential diagnosis.

SUGGESTED READINGS

1. Banwell B, Tenembaum S, Lennon VA, et al. Neuromyelitis optica-IgG in childhood inflammatory demyelinating CNS disorders. Neurology. 2008;70:344-52.
2. Barnett Y, Sutton IJ, Ghadiri M, et al. Conventional and advanced imaging in neuromyelitis optica. AJNR Am J Neuroradiol. 2014;35(8):1458-66.
3. Cobo Calvo A, Mañé Martínez MA, Alentorn-Palau A, et al. Idiopathic acute transverse myelitis: Outcome and conversion to multiple sclerosis in a large series. BMC Neurol. 2013;13:135.
4. Flanagan EP, McKeon A, Lennon VA, et al. Paraneoplastic isolated myelopathy: Clinical course and neuroimaging clues. Neurology. 2011;76:2089-95.
5. Flanagan EP, Weinshenker BG, Krecke KN, et al. Short myelitis lesions in aquaporin-4-IgG-positive neuromyelitis optica spectrum disorders. JAMA Neurol. 2015;72:81-7.
6. Flanagan EP, Weinshenker BG. Neuromyelitis optica spectrum disorders. Curr Neurol Neurosci Rep. 2014;14:483.
7. Hamid SHM, Elsone L, Mutch K, et al. The impact of 2015 neuromyelitis optica spectrum disorders criteria on diagnostic rates. Mult Scler. 2017;23(2):228-33.
8. Hamid SHM, Whittam D, Mutch K, et al. What proportion of AQP4-IgG-negative NMO spectrum disorder patients are MOG-IgG positive? A cross sectional study of 132 patients. J Neurol. 2017;264(10):2088-94.
9. Hyun JW, Jeong IH, Joung A, et al. Evaluation of the 2015 diagnostic criteria for neuromyelitis optica spectrum disorder. Neurology. 2016;86(19):1772-9.
10. Iype M, Kunju PAM, Saradakutty G, et al. Short term outcome of ADEM: Results from a retrospective cohort study from South India. Mult Scler Relat Disord. 2017;18:128-34.
11. Jarius S, Paul F, Franciotta D, et al. Cerebrospinal fluid findings in aquaporin-4 antibody positive neuromyelitis optica: Results from 211 lumbar punctures. J Neurol Sci. 2011;306:82-90.
12. Kitley J, Leite MI, Nakashima I, et al. Prognostic factors and disease course in aquaporin-4 antibody-positive patients with neuromyelitis optica spectrum disorder from the United Kingdom and Japan. Brain. 2012;135(6):1834-49.
13. Lannuzzi MC, Rybicki BA, Teirstein AS. Sarcoidosis. N Engl J Med. 2007;357(21):2153-65.
14. Leite MI, Coutinho E, Lana-Peixoto M, et al. Myasthenia gravis and neuromyelitis optica spectrum disorder: A multicenter study of 16 patients. Neurology. 2012;78:1601-7.
15. Mealy MA, Wingerchuk DM, Greenberg BM, et al. Epidemiology of neuromyelitis optica in the United States: A multicenter analysis. Arch Neurol. 2012;69(9):1176-80.
16. Miller DH, Leary SM. Primary-progressive multiple sclerosis. Lancet Neurol. 2007;6:903-12.
17. Polman CH, Reingold SC, Banwell B, et al. Diagnostic criteria for multiple sclerosis: 2010 revisions to the McDonald criteria. Ann Neurol. 2011;69:292-302.
18. Quek AM, McKeon A, Lennon VA, et al. Effects of age and sex on aquaporin-4 autoimmunity. Arch Neurol. 2012;69(8):1039-43.
19. Sato DK, Callegaro D, Lana-Peixoto MA, et al. Distinction between MOG antibody-positive and AQP4 antibody-positive NMO spectrum disorders. Neurology. 2014;82(6):474-81.
20. Sohn M, Culver DA, Judson MA, et al. Spinal cord neurosarcoidosis. Am J Med Sci. 2014;347:195-8.
21. Suzuki K, Nakamura T, Hashimoto K, et al. Hypothermia, hypotension, hypersomnia, and obesity associated with hypothalamic lesions in a patient positive for the anti-aquaporin 4 antibody: A case report and literature review. Arch Neurol. 2012;69(10):1355-9.
22. Takahashi T, Fujihara K, Nakashima I, et al. Anti-aquaporin-4antibody is involved in the pathogenesis of NMO: A study on antibody titre. Brain. 2007;130:1235-43.
23. Tanaka M, Tanaka K, Komori M, et al. Anti-aquaporin 4 antibody in Japanese multiple sclerosis: The presence of optic spinal multiple sclerosis without long spinal cord lesions and anti-aquaporin 4 antibody. J Neurol Neurosurg Psychiatry. 2007;78(9):990-2.
24. Titulaer MJ, Hoftberger R, Iizuka T, et al. Overlapping demyelinating syndromes and anti-N-methyl-D-aspartate receptor encephalitis. Ann Neurol. 2014;75:411-28.
25. Weinshenker BG, Wingerchuk DM. Neuromyelitis spectrum disorders. Mayo Clin Proc. 2017;92(4):663-79.
26. Wingerchuk DM, Banwell B, Bennett JL, et al. International consensus diagnostic criteria for neuromyelitis optica spectrum disorders. Neurology. 2015;85:177-189.
27. Wingerchuk DM, Hogancamp WF, O'Brien PC, et al. The clinical course of neuromyelitis optica (Devic's syndrome). Neurology. 1999;53(5):1107-14.
28. Wingerchuk DM, Lennon VA, Lucchinetti CF, et al. The spectrum of neuromyelitis optica. Lancet Neurol. 2007;6:805-15.
29. Wingerchuk DM. Neuromyelitis optica: Effect of gender. J Neurol Sci. 2009;286(1-2):18-23.

10
CHAPTER

Immune-mediated Neuropathies

Meena A Kanikannan, Sireesha Yareeda

INTRODUCTION

The immune-mediated neuropathies are a heterogeneous group of disorders with varied clinical presentations determined by the target and specificity of the immunologic attack. The immunologic process may be directed to either the peripheral nerves or the supporting blood vessels. Peripheral nerve myelin appears to be a frequent target, and a demyelinating neuropathy is the end result in many of these disorders. Vasculitic neuropathy, in which the pathologic process originates in the blood vessels and leads to nerve ischemia, results in a neuropathy characterized primarily by axonal loss.

CLINICAL CHARACTERISTICS OF IMMUNE-MEDIATED NEUROPATHIES

Our understanding of the immune-mediated polyneuropathies has grown dramatically over the past 20 years. It is known to comprise a heterogeneous set of disorders. They are currently classified as:
- Acute, e.g., Guillain–Barré syndrome (GBS) and occasionally vasculitic neuropathy
- Chronic, e.g., chronic immune-mediated demyelinating polyneuropathy (CIMDPs), neuropathy associated with systemic autoimmune diseases (vasculitic neuropathies, paraneoplastic neuropathies).

The characteristic features of inflammatory demyelinating neuropathy irrespective of time course are relatively symmetrical proximal dominant weakness in arms and legs with or without sensory disturbances, hyporeflexia or areflexia, and albuminocytological dissociation in cerebrospinal fluid (CSF). Demonstration of demyelination is required either on electrophysiology or nerve biopsy. In general, the electrodiagnostic features include—increased distal motor latency and proximal F-wave latency; decreased motor nerve conduction velocity; and excessive temporal dispersion and conduction block. Vasculitic neuropathy presents as painful mononeuritis or multifocal mononeuritis, or distal symmetrical axonal polyneuropathies.

Pathogenic mechanisms involve both antibody and cell-mediated immune responses. The immune response is built against the antigens located on the surface membrane of the axolemma (glycolipids, ion channels) and nuclear cytoplasm and against blood vessels in case of vasculitic neuropathy. Table 1 shows the autoantibodies in various autoimmune-mediated neuropathies. Antiganglioside antibodies are associated with GBS, multifocal

TABLE 1: Autoantibodies associated with autoimmune neuropathies

Antibody	Clinical features of associated neuropathy	Associated systemic disease
Antigangliosides	MMN, MND, GBS and variants	None
Sulfatide	Sensory-predominant neuropathy	None
Galopin (IgM kappa)	GALOP syndrome	None
Hu (ANNA-1)	SN autonomic and SMN	Small cell lung cancer (SCLC)
CV2/CRMP-5; amphiphysin; Ri (ANNA-2), ANNA-3; N-type CC	SMN	SCLC, thymoma, breast cancer
P-ANCA and C-ANCA	Painful mononeuritis multiplex; distal symmetric polyneuropathy less common	Churg–Strauss; polyarteritis nodosa; Wegener's granulomatosis
ANA; RF	Painful neuropathy; mononeuritis multiplex	Rheumatoid arthritis; systemic vasculitis
Ro/SSA; La/SSB	Painful sensory, predominantly small-fiber, neuropathy; sensory neuronopathy	Sjögren syndrome
Gliadin; endomysial; tTG	Mild distal sensory polyneuropathy	Celiac disease

ANA, antinuclear antibodies; ANCA, antineutrophil cytoplasmic antibodies; ANNA, antineuronal nuclear antibodies; CRMP, collapsin response mediator protein; MAG, myelin-associated glycoprotein; RF, rheumatoid factor; SGPG, sulfoglucuronyl glycosphingolipid; tTG, tissue transglutaminase; SN, sensory neuronopathy; SMN, sensory motor neuropathy; MMN, multifocal motor neuropathy; GBS, Guillain-Barré syndrome; MND, motor neuron disease; GALOP, gait ataxia with late onset polyneuropathy; CC, calcium channel; SSA, Sjögren's-syndrome-related antigen A, SSB, Sjögren's-syndrome-related antigen B.

motor neuropathy (MMN) and chronic ataxic neuropathy, ophthalmoplegia, monoclonal immunoglobulin (Ig) M protein, cold agglutinins and disialosyl antibodies (CANOMAD). Paranodal cell adhesion molecules like Neurofascin 155 (NF155), contactin 1 and contactin associated protein chronic inflammatory demyelinating polyneuropathy (CIDP) only] are the most consistent and clinically relevant targets in some CIDP and GBS patients. The antibodies against these antigens belong to IgG4 class, hence CIDP and GBS are considered as IgG4-related diseases.

Guillain–Barré Syndrome

The GBS is an acute self-limiting monophasic illness. It can affect individuals of all ages, but males are more often affected than females (1.5:1).

Pathogenesis

Host immune response to a preceding infection that cross-reacts with peripheral nerve components because of molecular mimicry forms the basis for the pathogenesis. Antibodies against glycolipids are present in 60% of the sera from GBS patients in acute phase. The role of these antiganglioside antibodies in the pathogenesis are established in some of the phenotypes (Table 2). They may be used as diagnostic markers of GBS. The immune

TABLE 2: Guillain-Barré syndrome variants and association of IgG antiganglioside antibodies with Guillain–Barré syndrome subtypes

Subtypes / variants	IgG antibodies against
Acute inflammatory demyelinating polyradiculoneuropathy	None
Acute motor axonal neuropathy	GM1 and GD1a
Acute motor and sensory axonal neuropathy	GM1 and GD1a
Acute motor conduction block neuropathy	GM1 and GD1a
Pharyngeal-cervical-brachial variant	GT1a (less frequently with GQ1b and GD1a)
Miller Fisher syndrome	GQ1b and GT1a
Acute ataxic neuropathy (without ophthalmoplegia)	GQ1b and GT1a
Pure sensory ataxic variant	GD1b (less frequently with GQ1b and GT1a)
Bickerstaff brainstem encephalitis	GQ1b and GT1a

response is directed towards the myelin or the axon of nerve, resulting in demyelinating and axonal forms of GBS. Most common infection is *Campylobacter jejuni* infection. Other infections like Cytomegalovirus, Epstein–Barr virus, and human immunodeficiency virus infection, *Mycoplasma pneumoniae*, influenza, varicella, and West Nile and Zika virus have also been associated with GBS. A small percentage of patients develop GBS after exposure to noninfectious triggers like immunization, surgery, trauma, and bone-marrow transplantation.

Clinical Features

Progressive (usually 2 weeks but not more than 4 weeks), mostly symmetric muscle weakness and global areflexia or hyporeflexia are the most essential clinical features of GBS. The weakness can vary from mild to severe, leading to nearly complete paralysis of all extremities, bifacial, respiratory and bulbar muscles. Symptoms usually start in the feet and typically spread proximally over the first few days. The original description was that of an "ascending" symmetrical paralysis described by Guillain, Barre´, and Strohl but there are exceptions to this. Neuropathic pain is common in GBS. Low back pain as well as radicular pain is described as, burning, prickly, and superficial pain. Mechanical ventilation is required in about 30%, and mild dysautonomia occurs in 70% of patients. There are several clinical and paraclinical factors predicting the need for mechanical ventilation but the most important bedside features are a combination of any two of the following features—single breath count, bulbar paresis and neck weakness. Red flags in the diagnosis of GBS are given in Box 1.

Guillain–Barré syndrome is a heterogeneous syndrome with several variants (Table 3). Most common types include acute inflammatory demyelinating polyneuropathy (AIDP) and acute motor axonal neuropathy. Acute motor and sensory axonal neuropathy and Miller Fisher syndrome are not very common. Acute inflammatory demyelinating polyneuropathy is the most common variant of GBS in most of the developed world and axonal forms are most common in Japan and China. In India, axonal forms and AIDP are equally seen.

Laboratory Diagnosis

Ancillary supportive tests include CSF analysis and electrophysiology. Cerebrospinal fluid evidence of albuminocytologic dissociation is found in 50–66% of patients with GBS after the first week of the onset of symptoms and in more than 75% of patients in the third week. Nerve conduction studies (NCS) are usually normal in the first week and they are diagnostic in second and third week of the onset of the disease. At least two sets of NCS are required to subtype GBS. There are several electrophysiological criteria to diagnose GBS but sensitivities vary. Most recently, new diagnostic criteria for all subtypes of GBS and their core clinical features were proposed by GBS classification group (Table 3). There are several conditions which mimic GBS which needs exclusion (Box 2).

Treatment

Intravenous immunoglobulins (IVIG) or plasma exchange (PE) is the standard treatment and both are equally effective. Combination therapy offers little benefit. Second course of IVIG may be offered in case of treatment failure, although this approach is based only on anecdotal experience. About 30% of patients develop neuromuscular respiratory failure and about 25% develop severe dysautonomia. Thus, supportive care with mechanical ventilation and intensive care unit management is extremely important to improve the survival. Mortality is 5% despite intensive care and most common causes include dysautonomia, pneumonia, and pulmonary thromboembolism. Approximately 5–10% of patients have a prolonged course with delayed and incomplete recovery.

Box 1: Red flags in diagnosis of Guillain–Barré syndrome

- Asymmetrical weakness
- Persistent bladder and bowel dysfunction
- Bladder or bowel dysfunction at onset
- More than 50 mononuclear leukocytes/mm^3 or presence of polymorphonuclear leukocytes in cerebrospinal fluid
- Distinct sensory level

TABLE 3: Diagnostic criteria for Guillain–Barré syndrome (GBS) and Miller Fisher syndrome and their subtypes

Classification	Core feature	Other salient features	Supportive investigations
Classic GBS	Symmetric pattern of weakness and areflexia in all four limbs including motor cranial nerves, progression of illness for up to 28 days after onset followed by a static state or improvement	Sensory symptoms or signs are usually mild, bilateral seventh cranial nerve involvement, autonomic dysfunction, absence of fever at onset, recovery beginning 2–4 week after progression ceases	Albuminocytological dissociation-elevated cerebrospinal fluid protein with less than 10 cells/μL; electrodiagnostic features of GBS
Bilateral facial weakness with paresthesia	Areflexia, no limb weakness, ataxia ocular nerve palsy	Some may have normal tendon reflexes, and no sensory symptoms	Electrophysiological evidence of neuropathy

Continued

Continued

Classification	Core feature	Other salient features	Supportive investigations
• Miller Fischer syndrome • Incomplete forms (absence of certain features or presence of single feature) • Bickerstaff's brainstem encephalitis (BBE) • Incomplete BBE	• Classically has ataxia, bilateral ophthalmoparesis and bilateral reduced or absent tendon reflexes • Acute ophthalmoparesis, acute ataxic neuropathy, acute ptosis, acute mydriasis • Hypersomnolence, ophthalmoplegia and ataxia. No weakness • Acute ataxic hypersomnolence	• No limb weakness • Monophasic illness pattern with the interval between onset and nadir of weakness between 12 hours and 28 days • Normal corticospinal tract involvement/ hypersomnolence –	• Albuminocytological dissociation-elevated cerebrospinal fluid protein with less than 10 cells/µL • Electrodiagnostic features are normal or indicate involvement of sensory nerves only • IgG antibodies against ganglioside GQ1b (present in about 85% of the patients)
Paraparetic GBS	• Oculomotor weakness with spreading of weakness to the extremities occurs in 50% of the patients • Presence of additional features of other variants • Overlap with Miller Fisher syndrome, overlap with acute ataxic neuropathy, overlap with BBE	• Electrodiagnostic features supportive of GBS • Presence of antiganglioside GQ1b/GT1a-IgG antibodies	• Albuminocytological dissociation-elevated cerebrospinal fluid protein with <10 cells/µL • Electrodiagnostic features supportive of GBS
• Pharyngo-cervico-brachial variant • Incomplete forms • Acute oropharyngeal, acute cervicobrachial	• Weakness involves pharyngeal, neck and upper limb muscles • No leg weakness • Progression of illness for up to 28 days after onset followed by a clinical plateau or improvement	–	–

> **Box 2: Differential diagnosis of Guillain–Barré syndrome**
>
> - Toxin induced neuropathy (hexacarbon abuse, lead, organophosphorus poisoning)
> - Porphyria
> - Recent diphtheria infection
> - Neuromuscular junction disorders (botulism, myasthenia gravis)
> - Metabolic myopathies (lipid storage myopathy, hypophosphatemia, hypokalemic paralysis)
> - Inflammatory myositis (dermatomyositis, viral myositis)
> - Hysterical paralysis
> - Tick paralysis
> - Basilar artery occlusion
> - Spinal cord compression
> - Transverse myelitis
> - Wernicke's syndrome and thiamine deficiency
> - Acute vasculitis

Chronic Immune-mediated Polyneuropathies

There are several heterogeneous entities that fall under the category:
- Chronic immune-mediated demyelinating polyneuropathies
- Immune-mediated neuropathies associated with systemic vasculitis
- Paraneoplastic neuropathies
- Neuropathies associated with other systemic diseases (infections, toxins, and drugs).

Chronic Immune-mediated Demyelinating Polyneuropathies

They include idiopathic CIDP (classical and atypical variants) and CIMDPs that are distinct from idiopathic CIDP. These are thought to result from different pathophysiological disease processes and have unique clinical and diagnostic characteristics with different treatment response but sharing the features of demyelination.

Pathogenesis

Both humoral and cell-mediated immune mechanisms are implicated in endoneurial inflammation and nerve demyelination in CIMDPs. The immunologic trigger of most forms of CIDP remains unclear but there is evidence to implicate injury mediated by complement pathways and antibodies directed against antigenic components of the myelin sheath. However, antibodies to NF155 or to contactin were detected in small numbers of patients with CIDP who had severe disease, in some cases associated with tremor. Neurofascin and contactin are critical structural elements of the paranodal loop attachment to the axolemma. These antibodies appear to target paranodal proteins and may disrupt the axonal-glial junctions, leading to nerve conduction slowing.

Whether CIMDP is a single disease or a syndrome is a debatable issue. There is a general agreement that CIMDPs other than idiopathic CIDP like MMN with conduction block; anti-myelin-associated glycoprotein (MAG) neuropathy; polyneuropathy associated with osteosclerotic multiple myeloma [with or without rest of polyneuropathy, organomegaly, endocrinopathy, monoclonal protein and skin changes (POEMS) syndrome] and CANOMAD are different from classic CIDP on the basis of clinical, electrodiagnostic, and therapeutic characteristics.

The CIMDPs present with one of the following clinical phenotypes and all share features of demyelination, inflammation and immune mediation.

Classic and Idiopathic Chronic Inflammatory Demyelinating Polyneuropathy

Multifocal acquired demyelinating sensory and motor neuropathy or Lewis–Sumner syndrome
- Chronic immune sensory polyradiculopathy
- Sensory-predominant CIDP
- Distal acquired demyelinating symmetric neuropathy
- Demyelinating neuropathy with central nervous system demyelination
- Gait ataxia with late onset polyneuropathy syndrome
- Pure motor neuropathy
- Multifocal motor neuropathy with conduction block
- Demyelinating neuropathy associated with systemic diseases (Table 4).

Clinical features of classic chronic inflammatory demyelinating polyneuropathy

The patients present either with an insidious onset of symmetrical progressive limb weakness involving proximal and distal muscles, sensory loss, and areflexia, or with a relapsing remitting course. Chronic inflammatory demyelinating polyneuropathy most commonly occurs in adults between the ages of 40 years and 60 years, but can affect the elderly and children. In one-third, the course is relapsing remitting especially in the young. Large-fiber sensory loss in the distal limbs is a common feature. Neuropathic pain is rare, occurring in only a minority of cases. Facial, oropharyngeal, and ocular involvement occurs in less than 15% of patients. The absence of atrophy in affected muscles is a feature in favor of CIDP. Autonomic dysfunction and ventilator failure develop in fewer than 10% of cases.

However, it can present with other clinical patterns based on regional and functional involvement (Table 5) still sharing the electrophysiological and CSF features. The clinical characteristic features are given in Table 6.

Occasionally, the initial manifestations of CIDP may have acute presentation mimicking GBS. Such cases can be reclassified as CIDP only after three or more relapses or progression of symptoms and signs beyond 9 weeks. This needs to be differentiated from treatment related fluctuations (TRFs) seen in GBS. Patients with TRF show transient improvement in power after receiving IVIG followed by deterioration within a time frame of 8 weeks.

Laboratory diagnosis

Diagnosis relies on clinical and electrophysiologic criteria and exclusion of other mimics (Table 4). The American Academy of Neurology (AAN) criteria is one such electrophysiological criteria used mostly for research purpose and the sensitivity is only 50–60%, whereas the European Federation of Neurological Societies-Peripheral Nerve Society criteria is most sensitive and specific for diagnosing CIDP. For the practicing clinician, these criteria should be taken in consideration with the clinical context. Cerebrospinal fluid studies, magnetic resonance imaging of roots and plexus is supportive (Fig. 1A). Neurosonology of peripheral nerves may be helpful and is inexpensive and convenient (Fig. 1B). The classic pathologic features of CIDP include demyelination, remyelination (onion bulbs), endoneurial edema, and inflammatory cell infiltrates in the epineurium and endoneurium. There is preferential involvement of the nerve roots. It is not mandatory to perform nerve biopsy in CIDP, it is helpful in those scenarios when CIDP is considered, but clinical and electrophysiological features are atypical or do not

TABLE 4: Chronic inflammatory demyelinating polyneuropathy-associated illnesses

Paraprotein associated disorders	• Monoclonal gammopathy of unknown significance • Osteosclerotic myeloma (POEMS syndrome)
Chronic infection	• Human immunodeficiency virus infection • Human T lymphotropic virus type 1 • Lyme disease • Hepatitis C • Cat scratch disease • Epstein–Barr infection
Systemic medical disorder	• Diabetes mellitus • Thyrotoxicosis • Chronic active hepatitis • Membranous glomerulonephropathy
Malignancy	• Hepatocellular carcinoma • Melanoma • Pancreatic carcinoma • Colon adenocarcinoma • Lymphoma • Paraneoplastic
Medications	• Interferon-alpha • Procainamide • Tacrolimus • Tumor necrosis factor antagonists
Other possible associations	• Vaccinations • Solid organ transplantation • Hereditary neuropathy (Charcot–Marie–Tooth disease)
Connective disorders tissue and autoimmune	• Systemic lupus erthematosus • Sjogren syndrome • Rheumatoid disease • Giant cell arteritis • Sarcoidosis • Inflammatory bowel disease

POEMS, Polyneuropathy, organomegaly, endocrinopathy, monoclonal plasma cell disorder, and skin changes.

fulfill accepted diagnostic criteria or when the differential diagnosis requires excluding the possibility of amyloidosis or vasculitis. The other laboratory tests performed are described in Table 4 and are to mainly exclude other causes.

The clinical features of CIMDPs other than idiopathic CIDP are given in Table 7.

Approach to CIMDPs is given in Flowchart 1.

Treatment

Steroids, PE and IVIG are the mainstay in the treatment of CIDP. Several regimes of steroid therapy are available in literature each having disadvantages and advantages. In patients refractory to these treatment modalities and also in case of steroid dependency and requiring long term maintenance therapy, other agents are used with variable

TABLE 5: Clinical phenotypes—chronic inflammatory demyelinating polyneuropathy (CIDP)

Classic CIDP	• Relapsing or progressive course >8 weeks • Generalized symmetric weakness; proximal>distal • Global hypo/areflexia • Distal large fiber sensory loss
Functional variants	• Pure motor • Pure sensory • Ataxic Chronic immune sensory polyradiculopathy
Regional variants	• Focal or multifocal CIDP • Multifocal acquired demyelinating sensory and motor • Lewis-Sumner syndrome • Upper limb pattern • Paraparetic • Distal acquired demyelinating symmetrical neuropathy) • Isolated cranial neuropathies

results (cyclophosphamide, mycophenolate, azathioprine, methotrexate, interferons, cyclosporine, tacrolimus). Patients with IgG4 related CIDP respond dramatically to rituximab. Alemtuzumab has been found to be useful in some patients with refractory CIDP.

Neuropathy with Systemic Vasculitis

Many systemic autoimmune diseases characterized by abnormal antibodies are associated with neuropathies. They include:
- Systemic vasculitides
  - Vasculitis associated with connective tissue diseases (Systemic lupus erythematosus)
  - Polyarteritis nodosa
  - Eosinophilic granulomatosis with polyangiitis (Churg–Strauss disease)
  - Wegener's granulomatosis.

Clinical Features

Vasculitis of peripheral nerves leads to multiple focal areas of ischemic injury. It is an important cause of axonal neuropathy and needs to be considered in almost any patient with a progressive axonal neuropathy. Certain nerves such as the common peroneal nerve and the ulnar nerve have a propensity for involvement by a vasculitic process probably due to their poor collateral supply.

The diagnosis should always be considered in patients presenting with a painful, asymmetric neuropathy (50%). Typically, a subacute presentation but sometimes a fulminant presentation can occur. One-third have a chronic, indolent course. Small fibers are rarely affected due to vasculitis. Exclusive motor or autonomic presentation is rare, 15% may have predominant sensory involvement and cranial nerve involvement occurs in only 10%. The signature phenotype is a mononeuropathy multiplex (35–65%). Distal symmetric neuropathy is also frequently observed.

TABLE 6: Clinical characteristics of chronic inflammatory demyelinating polyneuropathy (CIDP) phenotypes

Clinical characteristics	Chronic immune mediated demyelinating polyneuropathies					
	Chronic inflammatory demyelinating polyneuropathy	Pure motor chronic inflammatory demyelinating polyneuropathy	Chronic immune sensory polyradiculopathy	Distal acquired demyelinating sensory neuropathy	Ig4 antibody related chronic inflammatory demyelinating polyneuropathy	Multifocal acquired demyelinating sensory and motor neuropathy
Weakness	Symmetric; proximal + distal	Symmetric; proximal + distal	No or rarely mild weakness	Symmetric; distal only, mild or no weakness	• Severe, proximal >distal (NF155) • Aggressive onset, motor predominant, ataxia, tremor (anti-contactin 1 antibody)	• Asymmetric; distal > proximal • Upper limbs > lower limbs
Sensory deficits	Yes; symmetric	Absent	Yes, ataxia is early and prominent	Yes; symmetric	Ataxia and severe neuropathic pain (anti-CASPR antibody)	Yes; multifocal (distribution of individual nerves)
Reflexes	Reduced or absent symmetrically	Reduced or absent symmetrically	Reduced or absent	Reduced or absent symmetrically	Reduced or absent symmetrically	Reduced or absent (multifocal or diffuse)
Demyelinating features	Usually symmetric	Usually symmetric	Nerve biopsy may be normal	Usually symmetric; prolonged distal latencies	Mixed axonal and demyelinating	Asymmetric (multifocal)
Conduction block	Common	Common	Absent	Uncommon	Common	Common
Abnormal SNAPs	Usually symmetric	SNAPs are normal	SNAPs are normal	Usually symmetric	SNAPs are usually normal	Asymmetric
Cerebrospinal fluid protein	Usually elevated	Usually elevated	Usually elevated	Usually elevated	Usually elevated	Usually elevated

Continued

Immune-mediated Neuropathies

Continued

Clinical characteristics	Chronic inflammatory demyelinating polyneuropathy	Pure motor chronic inflammatory demyelinating polyneuropathy	Chronic immune sensory polyradiculopathy	Distal acquired demyelinating sensory neuropathy	IgG4 antibody related chronic inflammatory demyelinating polyneuropathy	Multifocal acquired demyelinating sensory and motor neuropathy
			Chronic immune mediated demyelinating polyneuropathies			
Monoclonal protein	Occasionally present, usually IgG or IgA	Rarely present Usually IgG or IgA	Rarely present, usually IgG or IgA	IgM-k present in the majority, 50–70% are MAG positive	Absent	Rarely present
Anti-GM1 antibodies	Rarely present	Absent	Absent	Not present	Anti-NF155 and CNTN-1 antibodies Anti-CASPR antibody	Rarely present
Treatment Response						
Steroids	Yes	Yes	Yes	Poor	Not very effective. Good Response to rituximab	Yes
IVIG	Yes	Better response with IVIG	Yes	Poor	Suboptimal response	Possible (more studies needed)
PE	Yes	Poor	Possible (more studies needed)	Poor	May respond	Yes

CIDP, chronic inflammatory demyelinating polyneuropathy; SNAP, sensory nerve action potential; NF155, neurofascin155; CASPR, contactin-associated protein; IVIG, intravenous immunoglobulin; PE, plasma exchange; CNTN-1, contactin 1.

Immune-mediated Neurological Disorders

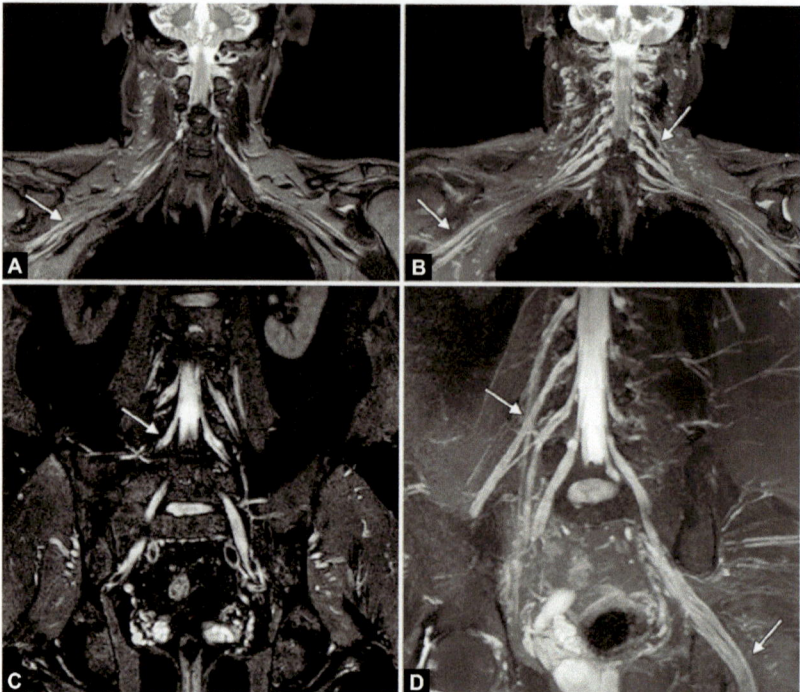

FIG. 1A: Magnetic resonance neurography of a 36-year-old female, disease duration of 2 years with remitting-relapsing course fulfilling European Federation of Neurological Societies-Peripheral Nerve Society criteria. The distribution of hypertrophy in typical chronic inflammatory demyelinating polyneuropathy is symmetric and predominant in the nerve roots.

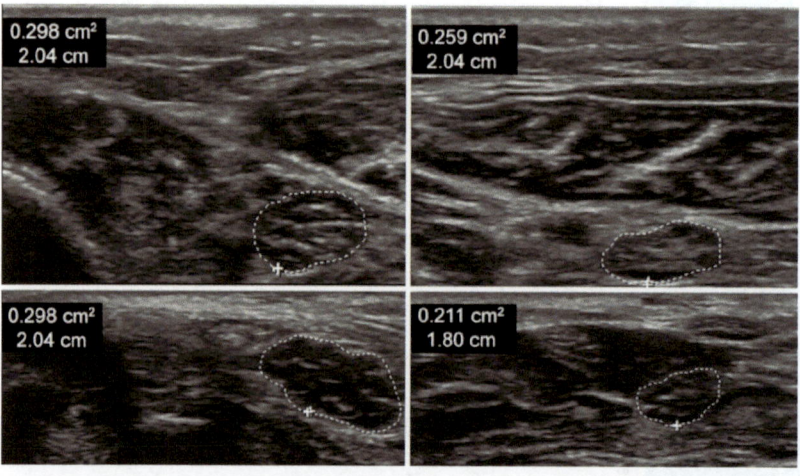

FIG. 1B: High-resolution ultrasonogram of right tibial and median nerve. Enlarged nerve and fascicles with preserved fascicular architecture and no abnormal color flow in a 38-year-old male with chronic inflammatory demyelinating polyneuropathy fulfilling European Federation of Neurological Societies-Peripheral Nerve Society criteria.

Immune-mediated Neuropathies

TABLE 7: Chronic immune-mediated demyelinating polyneuropathy other than chronic inflammatory demyelinating polyneuropathy (CIDP)

Syndrome	Monoclonal protein	Clinical phenotype	Electrodiagnostic studies	Treatment
POEMS (polyneuropathy, organomegaly, endocrinopathy, monoclonal plasma cell disorder, and skin changes)	IgG or IgA, lambda	Sensorimotor polyradiculoneuropathy (CIDP-like)	Demyelinating	• Patients with one to three bone lesions - radiation to the affected sites • Autologous peripheral blood stem cell transplantation - considered as a first-line treatment in patients with younger onset
CANOMAD (chronic ataxic neuropathy with ophthalmoparesis, M-protein, cold agglutinins, and disialosylganglioside antibodies)	• Cold agglutinins • Antibodies to GD1b/GQ1b	Chronic variant of MFS Chronic ataxic neuropathy with motor and small fiber preservation ophthalmoplegia, dysphagia, dysarthria	Demyelinating	Plasma exchange/IVIG

IgM paraproteinemic neuropathy (anti-MAG neuropathy)	Anti-MAG	Predominantly distal, chronic (duration over 6 months), slowly progressive, symmetric, predominantly sensory impairment, with ataxia, relatively mild or no weakness, and often tremor	• Disproportionately prolonged distal motor latency
			  ○ TLI≤0.25
			  ○ Uniform symmetrical reduction of conduction velocities; more severe sensory than motor involvement
			  ○ CB is very rare
				• Mild disease – symptomtic therapy
				• Significant chronic or progressive disability.
				• Immunosuppressive treatment may be considered, although none is of proven efficacy. IVIG or plasma exchange may be considered. In patients unresponsive to IVIG or plasma exchange), clinicians have used rituximab and cyclophosphamide

Continued

Continued

Syndrome	Monoclonal protein	Clinical phenotype	Electrodiagnostic studies	Treatment
Immunoglobulin M monoclonal gammopathy of undetermined significance	IgM kappa	Distal large fiber sensory predominant neuropathy with sensory ataxia	Demyelinating with prolonged distal latencies	Poor response to immunosuppressive therapy
Multifocal motor neuropathy	Anti-GM1 antibodies are frequently present	• Motor predominant; Asymmetric; distal >proximal; Upper limbs >lower limbs • Mild objective vibration sense deficits may be present	• Demyelinating with conduction block • SNAPs are normal	IVIG/Steroids

TLI: terminal latency index = distal conduction distance (mm)/[Conduction velocity (m/s) × distal motor latency (ms)]

MAG, myelin-associated glycoprotein; MFS, Miller Fisher syndrome; CB, conduction block; IVIG, intravenous immunoglobulin; SNAP, sensory nerve action potential.

Immune-mediated Neuropathies

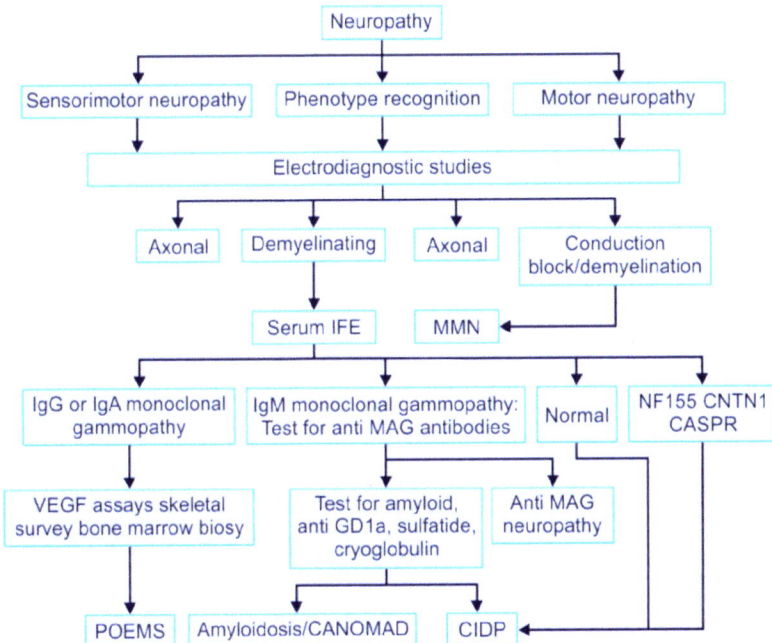

CIDP, chronic inflammatory demyelinating polyneuropathy; POEMS, polyneuropathy, organomegaly, endocrinopathy, monoclonal protein and skin changes; MAG, myelin-associated glycoprotein; MMN, multifocal motor neuropathy; IFE, immunofixation electrophoresis; VEGF, vascular endothelial growth factor; NF155, neurofascin 155; CNTV 1, contactin 1; CASPR, contactin associated protein; CANOMAD, chronic ataxic neuropathy, ophthalmoplegia, monoclonal immunoglobulin M protein, cold agglutinins and disialosyl antibodies.

FLOWCHART 1: Approach to chronic immune-mediated neuropathy.

An entity of nonsystemic vasculitic neuropathy is well recognized. These patients do not have clinical, laboratory, or pathologic evidence of organ involvement other than the peripheral nerves. They also do not have a connective tissue disease, malignancy, or another systemic inflammatory disease. Constitutional symptoms, if present, are mild, and erythrocyte sedimentation rate is usually only mildly elevated.

Others diseases like Sjögren syndrome and celiac disease cause immune-mediated nerve injury but not due to the primary vasculitis. The exact mechanisms are unclear. Sensory neuronopathy is commonly seen in Sjögren syndrome and celiac disease, but acute and chronic demyelinating neuropathies are also rarely associated with these syndromes. A causal relationship is not proven. Small fiber neuropathy presenting as painful, distal sensory symptoms is seen with Sjögren syndrome.

Laboratory Diagnosis

Laboratory evaluations are aimed at screening for systemic disease and organ involvement (serological studies). The definitive diagnosis of vasculitic neuropathy requires pathologic confirmation. The biopsy is preferably performed on a clinically or electrophysiologically involved sensory nerve. A possibly better approach is to perform a combined nerve and muscle biopsy of the superficial peroneal nerve (a sensory nerve) and the peroneus brevis muscle which increases the yield of the test. Histopathology of nerves shows perivascular inflammation mainly involving the epineural arteries with fibrinoid necrosis leading to thrombosis and ischemia (Fig. 2).

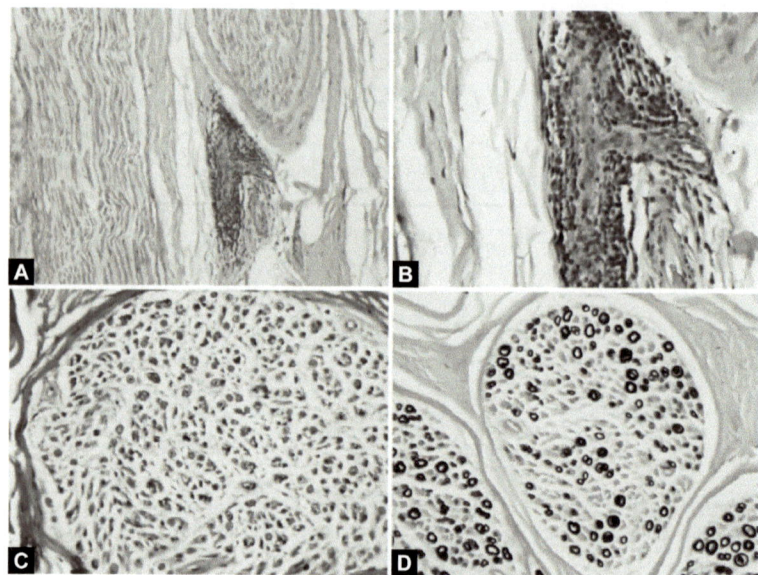

FIG. 2: A and **B,** Presence of perivascular lymphocytic infiltrate with vascular wall destruction; **C,** Increase in endoneurial collagen (MTX40 **D,** Sectorial multifocal nonuniform fiber loss (KpalX40). *(For color version, see plate 2)*

Treatment

Treatment options include steroids and other steroid sparing immunosuppressives (cyclophosphamide, methotrexate, azathioprine, and mycophenolate mofetil). More recently, rituximab and IVIG have been tried with some success. Nonsystemic vasculitic neuropathy tends to be less aggressive and less disabling than systemic vasculitic neuropathy. The Peripheral Nerve Society task force recommended starting with corticosteroid monotherapy unless the neuropathy is rapidly progressive, although many patients still require combination therapy with a cytotoxic agent to maintain remission.

Paraneoplastic Neuropathies

These are rare syndromes occurring in isolation or as a constellation of neurological manifestations with simultaneous involvement of other sites in the neuroaxis. Phenotypic presentations include sensory neuronopathy, autonomic enteric neuropathy, demyelinating neuropathy and motor neuropathy. Paraneoplastic sensorimotor neuropathy may manifest as a length-dependent neuropathy, indistinguishable from other common types of axonal polyneuropathy or, less commonly, as a mononeuropathy multiplex pattern resembling vasculitic neuropathy. They typically precede the cancer (lung, breast, colon, and thymus) when the tumor burden is less. It is postulated that the malignancy serves as a stimulus for the immune system to mount an immune response involving both cell-mediated and humoral components with the target antigen falling into one of the two categories (anti-nuclear or cytoplasmic antibodies and anti-surface ion channel antibodies). Anti-Hu and anti-CV2/collapsin response mediator protein 5 are frequently associated with paraneoplastic neuropathy. Diagnosis is supported by serology with commercial assays available that can detect these antibodies in CSF and serum. Cerebrospinal fluid examination is nonspecific and if the suspicion is high based on clinical presentation or antibody results, a fluorodeoxyglucose-positron emission tomography should be performed. Even if malignancy is not found in a high-risk individual, it is mandatory to repeat cancer screening studies every 3-6 months for several years. As these syndromes are rare, treatment guidelines have not been formulated. Commonly used immunomodulatory therapies include IVIG, intravenous or oral corticosteroids, PE, rituximab, and cyclophosphamide; however, the most important therapeutic intervention to prevent progression of neuropathy is to treat the underlying malignancy with the expectation; this will prevent further progression of neuropathy.

CONCLUSION

- Immune-mediated neuropathies are heterogeneous entity and are broadly classified based on a time frame into acute disorders such as GBS and, occassionally, vasculitic neuropathy and chronic neuropathy such as CIMDP, neuropathy associated with systemic diseases, vasculitic and paraneoplastic disorders
- Clinically, demyelinating neuropathies are characterized by symmetrical, proximal motor weakness with or without sensory loss, areflexia or hyporeflexia
- Classical CIDP is distinct from MMN with conduction block, anti-MAG associated neuropathy, POEMS and CANOMAD; and all of them fall under the rubric of CIMDPs
- The prototypic presentation of vasculitic neuropathy is mononeuropathy multiplex
- Paraneoplastic neuropathy typically precedes cancer and serves as a marker for their early detection when the tumor burden is less
- Steroids, IVIG and PE are the mainstay of the treatment. Maintenance therapy includes long-term treatment with immunosuppressive drugs.

SUGGESTED READINGS

1. Alexander M, Prabhakar AT, Aaron S, et al. Utility of neurophysiological criteria in Guillain Barre' syndrome: Subtype spectrum from a tertiary referral hospital in India. Neurol India. 2011;59:722-6.
2. Devaux JJ, Miura Y, Fukami Y, et al. Neurofascin-155 IgG4 in chronic inflammatory demyelinating polyneuropathy. Neurology. 2016;86:800-7.
3. Kalita J, Kumar M, Misra UK. Prospective comparison of acute motor axonal neuropathy and acute inflammatory demyelinating polyradiculoneuropathy in 140 children with Guillain-Barré syndrome in India. Muscle Nerve. 2018 May;57(5):761-5.
4. Kalita J, Misra UK, Goyal G, et al. Guillain-Barré syndrome: Subtypes and predictors of outcome from India. J Peripher Nerv Syst. 2014;19(1):36-43.
5. Kannan Kanikannan MA, Durga P, Venigalla NK, et al. Simple bedside predictors of mechanical ventilation in patients with Guillain-Barre syndrome. J Crit Care. 2014;29(2):219-23.
6. Kannan MA, Ch RK, Jabeen SA, et al. Clinical, electrophysiological subtypes and antiganglioside antibodies in childhood Guillain-Barré syndrome. Neurol India. 2011;59:727-32.
7. Miura Y, Devaux JJ, Fukami Y, et al. Contactin 1 IgG4 associates to chronic inflammatory demyelinating polyneuropathy with sensory ataxia. Brain. 2015;138:1484-91.
8. Murthy J, Sundram C, Meena AK, et al. Vasculitic neuropathy: Clinical electrophysiological and histopathological characteristics. 1998;46(1):18-22.
9. Querol L, Nogales-Gadea G, Rojas-Garcia R, et al. Antibodies to contactin-1 in chronic inflammatory demyelinating polyneuropathy. Ann Neurol. 2013;73(3):370-80.
10. Querol L, Nogales-Gadea G, Rojas-Garcia R, et al. Neurofascin IgG4 antibodies in CIDP associate with disabling tremor and poor response to IVIg.AU Neurology. 2014;82(10):879-86.
11. Van den Bergh PY, Hadden RD, Bouche P, et al. European Federation of Neurological Societies/Peripheral Nerve Society guideline on management of chronic inflammatory demyelinating polyradiculoneuropathy: Report of a joint task force of the European Federation of Neurological Societies and the Peripheral Nerve Society—first revision. Eur J Neurol. 2010;17(3):356-63.
12. Wakerley BR, Uncini A, Yuki N, et al. Guillain-Barré and Miller Fisher syndromes—new diagnostic classification. Nat Rev Neurol. 2014;10(9):537-44.

CHAPTER 11

Autoimmune Disorders of the Neuromuscular Junction

*Sarala Govindarajan, Harish Jayakumar, Yashodara Priyadarshini,
Lakshmi Narasimhan Ranganathan, Sindhuja Lakshminarasimhan, Tushar VP*

INTRODUCTION

Myasthenia gravis (MG) is an autoimmune disorder of the neuromuscular junction (NMJ) causing severe neurological impairment which is often reversible. The mechanism of NMJ failure could be destruction of the normal structures responsible for efficient functioning and transmission of signal or impairment or dysfunctional activity of the same due to targeted mutations as observed in congenital myasthenic syndromes. In most patients, NMJ failure is due to antibodies directed against the NMJ acetylcholine receptor (AChR). In patients where the antibodies are not to be found, sites other than AChR are implicated. For a better understanding of the autoimmune neuromuscular disorders, the various targets of autoimmune attack need to be identified.

NORMAL PHYSIOLOGY AND ANTIGENIC TARGETS

As soon as the action potential arrives at the nerve terminal, the vesicles containing ACh reach the terminal end near the synaptic cleft. The vesicles fuse with the membrane to release the ACh into the cleft. During development, a heparin sulphate proteoglycan, agrin is released from the nerve terminal. It fuses with the low-density lipoprotein receptor-related protein 4 (LRP4). This facilitates activation of muscle-specific tyrosine kinase (MuSK). Activated MuSK then binds to the phosphotyrosine-binding domain of adaptor protein—DOK7 (downstream-of-kinase or docking-protein 7). It belongs to a family of cytoplasmic signaling adaptor proteins that includes DOK1-7 and is a muscle intrinsic activator of MuSK which further stimulates dimerization and transphosphorylation of the activation loop of MuSK. This leads to AChR clustering at the site of release. Thus, agrin, MuSK, and LRP4 are crucial in clustering of AChR (Fig. 1).

Autoimmune neuromuscular disorders can be classified into the following groups (Flowchart 1):
- Presynaptic
  - Voltage-gated calcium channels (VGCC)
  - Anti SOX-1 antibodies.
- Postsynaptic
  - Anti-AChR antibodies
  - Anti-MuSK antibodies
  - Antibodies to non-AChR NMJ proteins
  - Autoantibodies directed against non-AChR skeletal muscle proteins.

Autoimmune Disorders of the Neuromuscular Junction

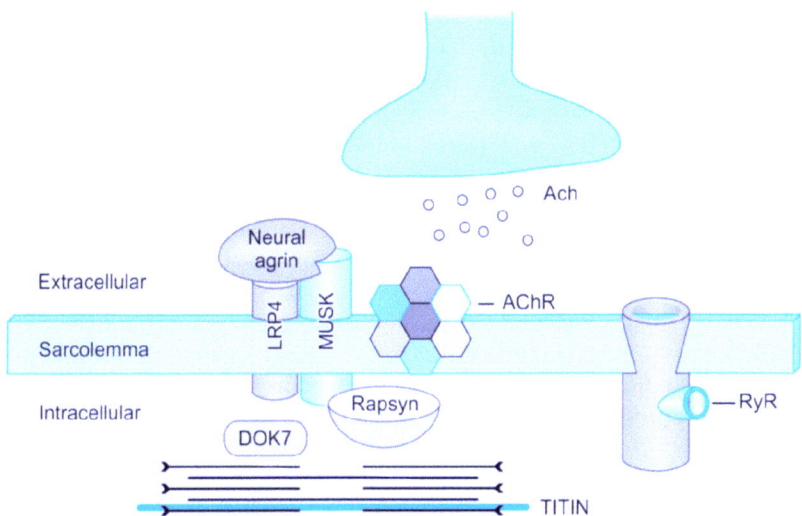

ACHR, acetylcholine receptor; MuSK, muscle-specific tyrosine kinase; LRP, low-density lipoprotein receptor-related protein; RyR, ryanodine receptor; DOK7, downstream of tyrosine kinase 7.

FIG. 1: Normal physiological process in the neuromuscular junction and potential antigenic targets.

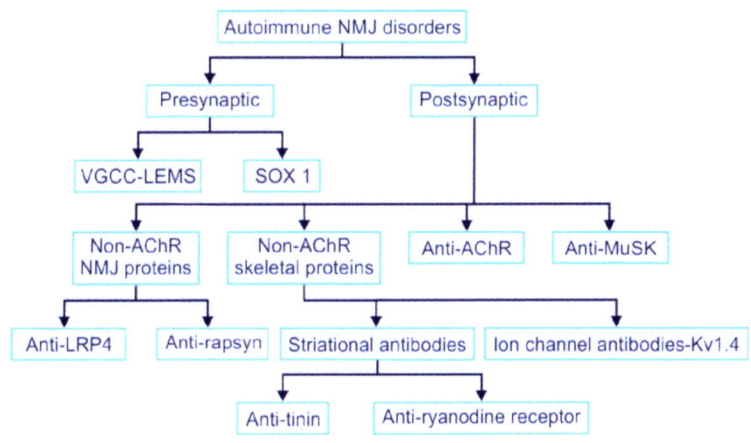

NMJ, neuromuscular junction; VGCC, voltage-gated calcium channels; LEMS, Lambert–Eaton myasthenic syndrome; AChR, acetylcholine receptor; MuSK, muscle-specific tyrosine kinase; LRP, low-density lipoprotein receptor-related protein.

FLOWCHART 1: Classification of autoimmune neuromuscular junction disorders.

Presyaptic Antibodies

Voltage-gated Calcium Channels—Lambert–Eaton Myasthenic Syndrome

Incidence

Lambert–Eaton myasthenic syndrome (LEMS) is an uncommon condition seen predominantly in elderly population. Around 50% have malignancy association of which

40% have small cell lung cancer (SCLC). Of the total, 3% of SCLC have LEMS. Other malignant conditions associated are Hodgkin's lymphoma, malignant thymoma and atypical carcinoid syndromes. In the remaining population without malignancy, 27% have autoimmune disorders like type 1 diabetes mellitus or hypothyroidism. A positive family history can also be obtained in patients with autoimmune association. An overlap syndrome with MG has been reported.

Pathophysiology

Antibodies are present which are directed against the VGCC in the presynaptic nerve terminal thereby interfering with the presynaptic calcium influx required for ACh release. P/Q type (95%), L type and N type are the most important channels affected. In paraneoplastic LEMS, the functional VGCC in the surface membrane of SCLC probably explains the reason for abnormal antibody production while it can be attributed to abnormal antibody production in autoimmune LEMS.

Clinical Features

Typically presents with slowly progressive proximal muscle weakness predominantly of lower limbs along with autonomic dysfunction in the form of dry mouth, erectile dysfunction, blurring of vision and constipation. Cranial nerve symptoms, though possible are less common than MG. Acute presentation can be in the form of respiratory failure. On examination, they have weakness predominantly of hip girdle muscles with diminished deep tendon reflexes. This improves typically with maximal isometric contraction of about 10 seconds and is called postsynaptic or postexercise facilitation. A paradoxical eyelid elevation can be seen after sustained up gaze which helps in differentiating from fatiguable ptosis of MG.

Diagnosis

Lambert–Eaton myasthenic syndrome is diagnosed on the basis of a combination of clinical features with supportive electrophysiology and presence of VGCC antibodies. Radioimmunoassay can detect antibodies against P/Q type channels in 85–95% cases and against N type VGCC in 30–40% cases. Electrophysiology studies show decreased baseline compound muscle action potential amplitude which increases and shows an incremental response following high frequency repetitive nerve stimulation or brief maximal isometric contraction of 10 seconds called postexercise facilitation. Single fiber electromyography shows significant jitter with transmission block improving with high firing rates.

Treatment

The basic approach would be to look for a primary underlying malignancy like squamous cell carcinoma. Medications like guanidine, aminopyridines, pyridostigmine and intravenous immunoglobulin (IVIG) have all been used with varying success. Immunosuppressive agents like prednisolone with azathioprine or plasmapheresis have been used in long term.

Prognosis

The prognosis is guarded and determined by the underlying condition severity, malignancy or autoimmune and the severity of weakness. Medicines provide only partial symptom relief and exacerbations can be seen during periods of illness or use of medications that impair neuromuscular transmission. Death usually is from the underlying malignancy.

Anti-SOX-1 Antibodies

Another presynaptic antibody whose pathogenic role is unclear is against—"SRY-like high-mobility-group box"—SOX-1 proteins. Initially, they were recognized as autoantibodies directed against Bergmann glia, a specialized cell type found in the cerebellum, which were later identified to be SOX-1 proteins. They are considered as anti-glial nuclear antibody. Anti-SOX-1 antibodies are implicated in paraneoplastic LEMS and paraneoplastic neuropathy. This antibody is positive in 67% of SCLC–LEMS patients, 22–32% of patients with SCLC without LEMS and only in 5% of nontumor LEMS patients.

Postsynaptic Antibodies

Anti-AChR Antibodies-Myasthenia Gravis

Myasthenia gravis is the most common immune-mediated disorder of the NMJ. Incidence of myasthenia ranges from 9 to 30 per million. There is a female preponderance in the first 5 decades of life while men are more commonly affected after 50 years of age. Ocular myasthenia is common in juvenile age group and MuSK myasthenia is frequent in younger women.

Pathophysiology

Acetylcholine receptor antibodies are seen in up to 85% of patients with generalized myasthenia and 50% with ocular myasthenia. Other antibodies associated with myasthenia are MuSK, LRP4, agrin and cortactin. AChR antibodies are IgG1 or IgG3 humoral autoimmune response directed against muscle nicotinic AChR-α leading to endplate AChR loss, simplification of the postsynaptic membrane and derangement of neuromuscular transmission (Fig. 2). Three types of AChR antibodies are recognized:
1. Binding (Fig. 3)
2. Blocking (Fig. 4)
3. Modulating (Fig. 5).

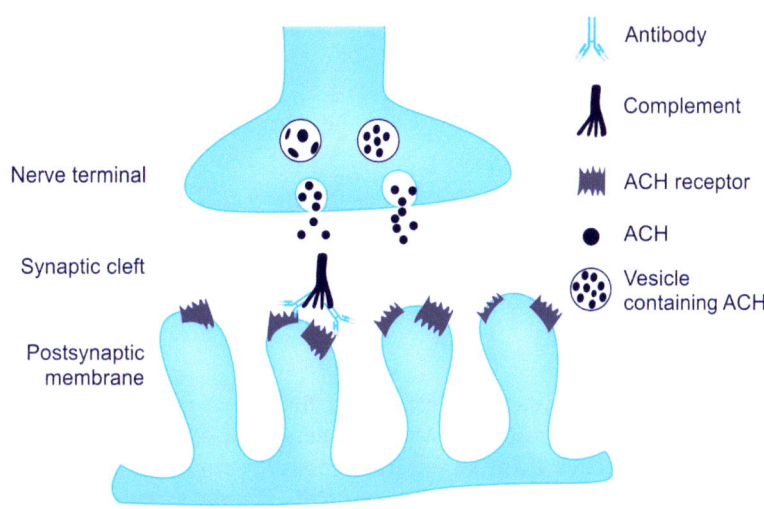

ACh, acetylcholine.
FIG. 2: Antibody binding resulting in complement activation.

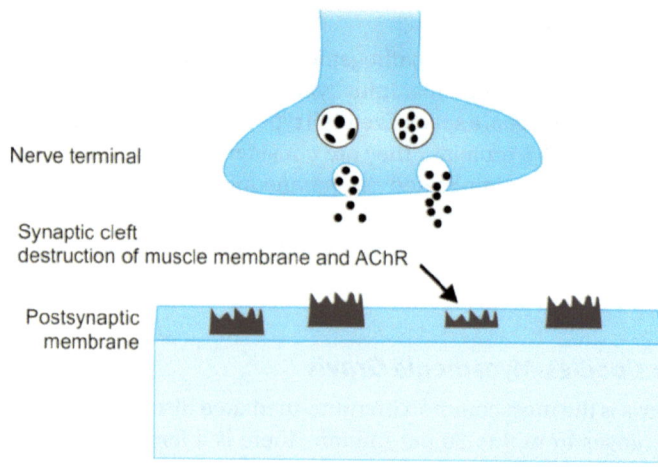

AChR, acetylcholine receptor.

FIG. 3: Destruction and focal lysis of the postsynaptic folds at the neuromuscular junction leading to the reduction of acetylcholine receptor and acetylcholine-related at the end-plate.

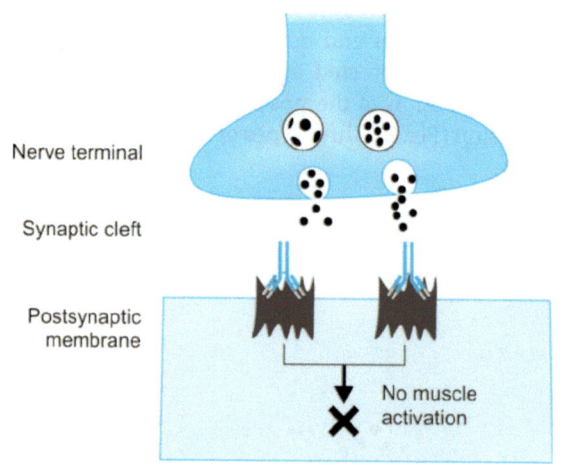

AChR, acetylcholine receptor.

FIG. 4: Blocking of acetylcholine receptor is pathologically important in acute exacerbations of myasthenia, usually present along with binding antibodies. Blocking antibodies correlate with the severity of the weakness.

Clinical Features

Ocular involvement is the initial manifestation in 50–60% of patients though many of them develop generalized myasthenia within 3 years of onset. Approximately 15–25% continue to have only ocular involvement throughout the course of illness. Fatigability and fluctuating weakness is the hallmark feature of MG. Diurnal variation with worsening towards the end of the day is also a distinguishing feature. Ocular involvement causes ptosis and diplopia. Ptosis can be unilateral or bilateral asymmetric. Manual elevation of the

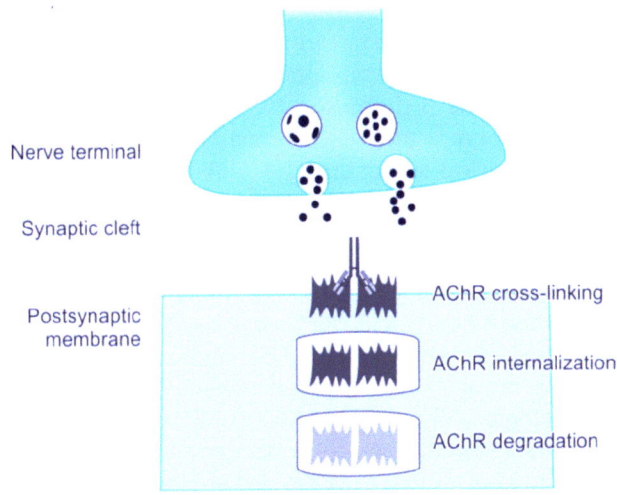

MG, myasthenia gravis; AChR, acetylcholine receptor.

FIG. 5: Modulating antibodies bind to acetylcholine receptor and causes cross linking, which subsequently leads to their internalization and degradation. High levels of modulating antibodies are seen in thymomatous myasthenia gravis.

ptotic eye causes ptosis of the opposite eye (curtain sign). Sustained lateral gaze or upgaze resulting in extraocular muscle weakness can elicit diplopia within 15–30 seconds. Pupils are usually spared. Pseudointernuclear opthalmoplegia may be seen. Other ocular signs include ocular quiver, Cogan's lid twitch sign, and frontalis overactivity. Facial muscles are frequently involved. Bulbar weakness causes dysphagia and regurgitation of feeds. Fatiguable weakness of chewing and jaw drop due to weak jaw closure is also suggestive of myasthenia. Weakness of both neck flexors and extensors can occur with flexor weakness being more common. Orthopnea may occur due to diaphragmatic weakness. Limb involvement causes proximal extremity weakness with arm weakness more common than lower limb weakness. Less commonly distal or asymmetric weakness can occur. Patient may be unaware of proximal weakness and it can be brought out on examination. Deltoid, triceps and hip flexors can be easily assessed for fatiguable weakness. Single breath count is useful in assessing for respiratory involvement and fatigable dysarthria. Quantitative MG test score incorporates ocular, bulbar, respiratory and proximal muscle strength and can be used to assess severity and response to treatment. Clinically, myasthenia is classified into five stages according to Myasthenia Gravis Foundation of America classification. Infections and certain drugs like neuromuscular blocking agents and aminoglycosides can precipitate myasthenic crisis which is a life-threatening emergency.

Of total, 50–80% of AChR positive patients have thymic hyperplasia while thymoma is detected in 10–20% of patients with myasthenia.

Diagnosis
- Ice pack test: Crushed ice in a plastic bag is placed over the ptotic eye for 2–5 minutes, and eyelid positions before and after application of ice pack are compared
- Edrophonium test: Edrophonium is administered intravenously and improvement in ptosis and extraocular weakness is looked for. It has a sensitivity of 71–95% for diagnosis of myasthenia

- Electrophysiological tests: Repetitive nerve stimulation can be done in nasalis, orbicularis oculi, trapezius, deltoid, and forearm muscles. Sensitivity is 75% in generalized myasthenia and 50% in ocular form. Approximately 10% decrement between first and fifth muscle potentials is diagnostic. Single fiber electromyography is highly sensitive for diagnosis of myasthenia. Abnormal jitter is seen in 95–99% of patients with myasthenia. Serological testing includes antibodies to AChR, MuSK and LRP4. Computed tomography (CT) chest is necessary to rule out thymoma.

Management

Pyridostigmine inhibits acetylcholinesterase at the NMJ and increases the availability of ACh. It is started at 30 mg 4 hourly and can be increased to 60 mg every 4 hours. Low dose prednisolone is useful for ocular and mild generalized myasthenia. Steroid sparing agents include azathioprine and mycophenolate mofetil. Myasthenic crisis is managed with mechanical ventilation, IVIG or plasmapheresis. Rituximab is effective in refractory myasthenia. Patients with thymoma require thymectomy. Education of patients is crucial and they should be given a list of drugs to be avoided in myasthenia.

Anti-MuSK Antibodies

Muscle-specific tyrosine kinase-myasthenia gravis (MuSK-MG) may present with atypical features distinct from myasthenia. When considered as a group, there exists significant clinical differences between groups of AChR myasthenia and MuSK myasthenia. However, significant overlap tends to occur between both, making it difficult to make an exact diagnosis.

Pathophysiology

Anti-MuSK antibodies belong to IgG4 class of antibodies. MuSK antibodies tend to bind with the N-terminal half of the extracellular domain of MuSK, thereby functionally inhibiting agrin-induced AChR clustering. Significant inhibition leads to dispersion of AChR and subsequently end plate dispersion. Muscle-specific tyrosine kinase antibodies have been proposed to have a presynaptic as well as postsynaptic effect on NMJ transmission. The disease process is not complement mediated. Studies have also demonstrated that anti-MuSK IgG tends to target the MuSK-ColQ (Collagen Q tail of anticholinesterase) and thereby interfering with the binding of MuSK to collagen tail. Thymus does not appear to have a role in the pathogenesis of MuSK-MG.

Clinical Features

Disease onset tends to be much earlier, in general the third or the fourth decade. There is female predominance, although exclusivity has not been demonstrated. Clinical features are usually atypical such as selective facial, bulbar, neck, shoulder and respiratory muscle weakness with substantial muscle atrophy, infrequently with relative sparing of ocular muscles. Respiratory crises tend to be more common. Fatiguable weakness, though significant, will be difficult to demonstrate in patients as the muscle weakness will be severe at presentation. Most patients tend to become worse with angiotensin-converting-enzyme inhibitors (ACEIs) and may have profuse fasciculations.

Diagnosis

Diagnosis is by identification of antibodies in the serum. It is seen in 50% of the patients with generalized myasthenia who lack AChR antibodies. Anti-MuSK antibodies seem to correlate with the disease severity and also with the response to immunotherapy. Anti-MuSK IgG4 may therefore serve as a good biological marker of the disease. False positive cases have not been reported and anti-MuSK antibodies are very rarely found in association with anti-AChR antibodies.

Management

Muscle-specific tyrosine kinase myasthenia responds poorly to ACEIs. They respond well to corticosteroids and steroid-sparing agents, though most patients remain dependent on steroids despite concomitant therapy with steroid-sparing agents. Also, the patients respond very well to plasma exchange, while IVIG is less effective. Rituximab should be considered in cases with poor response to initial immunotherapy.

Double-seronegative Myasthenia Gravis

Sometimes, approximately 7–8% patients with clinical features of MG will have neither anti-AChR nor anti-MuSK antibodies. In such patients, "low affinity" anti-AChR antibodies should be looked out for. Their action is complement mediated.

Antibodies to Nonacetylcholine Receptor Neuromuscular Junction Proteins

Proteins that are a part of NMJ and are being recently diagnosed to be potential targets include LRP4 and Rapsyn. Though, their defective production or deficiency can result in congenital myasthenic diseases, increasing evidence points towards them being a potential target and also a cause of double-seronegative MG.

LRP4 Antibodies

Lipoprotein receptor related protein 4 is a member of the low-density lipoprotein receptor-related protein family of transmembrane proteins. Lipoprotein receptor related protein 4 is expressed by subsynaptic myonuclei in the postsynaptic membrane. It binds with agrin and subsequently activates MuSK. It activates an intracellular signaling cascade leading to aggregation of AChR, as explained previously.

Pathophysiology

Anti-LRP4 antibodies alter the interaction between agrin-LRP4 and may significantly alter the agrin signaling pathway, thereby reducing AChR clustering. Though, LRP4 defects at the time of NMJ development have shown to be symptomatic, the effects of LRP4 antibodies in a mature developed muscle is not yet fully understood. Two different mechanisms have been postulated:
1. Complement mediated destruction of motor end plate
2. Defective aggregation of AChR. Lipoprotein receptor related protein 4 belongs to IgG1 subclass, and their effects are complement mediated.

Clinical Features

The occurrence of anti-LRP4 antibodies have a female predominance with mean age of onset to be 46.5 years. They tend to present with moderate to severe weakness at onset. Symptoms of weakness tend to predominate in facial and bulbar muscles (86%), neck weakness (86%), limb weakness (71%), ocular weakness (50%), and dyspnea (29%). These antibodies were found in 9.2% of patients with double-seronegative MG, but not in anti-AChR or anti-MuSK positive patients. These antibodies were found to be specific for MG, as they were not demonstrated in patients with other neurological or psychiatric illness as in other antibodies.

Management

All patients were shown to improve with a combination of ACEI and two or more forms of immunotherapy (corticosteroids and immunosuppressive therapy—azathioprine, IVIG). A small cohort who received this combination had demonstrated complete stable remission, with or without minimal symptoms.

Anti-Rapsyn Antibodies

Rapsyn is an intracellular end plate protein that is essential for the aggregation and clustering of AChR at the postsynaptic membrane. It is a cytoplasmic 43-kDa protein present on the inner aspect of the cell membrane which binds noncovalently with the beta subunit of the AChR. It has been postulated that immune-mediated anti-Rapsyn attack may contribute to the pathogenicity in MG. It has been found in 15% of patients with MG. Anti-Rapsyn antibodies were demonstrated most commonly in thymomatous MG. The pathogenicity and its role in producing MG is questionable as it is also present in other autoimmune diseases like lupus, and also seen in procainamide-induced myopathy.

Autoantibodies Directed Against Nonacetylcholine Receptor Skeletal Muscle Proteins

Antibodies against non-AChR muscle proteins can be subdivided into skeletal muscle proteins and non-AChR ion channels. The antibodies directed against proteins in skeletal muscle also includes striated muscle intracellular proteins—actin, myosin, titin and ryanodine receptor (RyR). Since, these are intracellular, these targets are not directly accessible to autoantibodies. This would imply that these antibodies are not pathogenic. However, evidence has shown their presence and correlation with disease severity in MG indicating that they may cause weakness through unknown mechanisms. Striational antibodies may occur in other autoimmune diseases and also in patients with thymoma without MG. Striational antibodies are reflective of thymic pathology and are most commonly suspected in patients with onset before the age of 40 years, but they also tend to occur more commonly in older patients with more severe disease and also along with anti-AChR antibodies. The major targets include titin and RyR.

Anti-titin Antibodies

Titin, an intracellular 3,000 kDa protein, is the largest known protein with length of 1 μm stretching throughout the sarcomere. It is one of the major antigenic targets in MG. Antibodies to titin belong to IgG1 subclass and therefore complement mediated attack is implicated. They tend to present with more severe disease. Patients present with a severe muscle disease because coexistent myopathy has also been observed. Titin is expressed in thymomatous tissue. Anti-titin antibodies are seen in 70–90% patients with thymoma and 50% of patients with late onset MG without thymoma. Almost 95% of patients with thymomatous MG have anti-titin antibodies, which makes anti-titin antibody assay as sensitive as CT chest. Hence, any patient presenting with a combination of muscle pain, elevated creatine phosphokinase and features of myasthenia should always be evaluated for the presence of thymoma and anti-titin antibodies. It is also shown that anti-titin antibodies correlate with disease severity. They are more likely to be refractive to therapy. Anti-titin antibodies are also seen rarely in early onset MG, AChR antibody-positive patients, but not reported to be positive in double-seronegative or MuSK MG.

Anti-ryanodine Receptor Antibodies

Ryanodine receptor is a calcium channel of the sarcoplasmic reticulum. There are three different types of ryanodine receptors i.e. RyR1, RyR2 and RyR3, which are primarily expressed in skeletal muscle, cardiac muscle, and brain, respectively. The primary function of the RyR is the opening and release of calcium ions into the sarcoplasmic reticulum which is an essential step in excitation contraction coupling. Ryanodine receptor antibodies belong to IgG1 or IgG3 subclass and therefore can activate complement and inhibit release of calcium into the reticulum. The combination of anti-titin antibodies and anti-RyR antibodies is 95% sensitive and 70% specific for thymoma. Ryanodine receptor antibodies can bind to both skeletal and cardiac muscle receptor. They can cause myositis and myocarditis as well. Hence, in patients presenting with myasthenia, muscle pain, palpitations, arrhythmias, and sudden death should alert the possibility of Ryanodine receptor antibodies antibody myasthenia. RyR are strongly associated with invasive or malignant thymoma and therefore presence of RyR antibodies after thymectomy should raise suspicion of residual thymomatous tissue and should prompt for re-exploration.

Antibodies Against Nonacetylcholine Receptor Ion Channels

Antibodies against α-subunit of voltage-gated potassium channel Kv1.4 is implicated to cause MG in approximately 12–28% of Japanese patients. They tend to present with bulbar symptoms, myasthenic crisis and myocarditis. Patients may be observed to have palpitations, prolonged QT interval, and elevated cardiac enzymes. Anti-Kv1.4 antibodies were demonstrated in patients with bulbar symptoms in Japanese patients and ocular symptoms in Caucasian patients. They do not present with clinical or electrophysiological evidence of neuromyotonia because they are directed against muscle potassium channel Kv1.4, rather than neuronal potassium channel Kv1.1 as seen in neuromyotonia. They have a favorable response to calcineurin inhibitors.

CONCLUSION

Myasthenia is increasingly being considered as a disease spectrum with wide variety of presentation and it is not fair to restrict the disease process to just AChR and MuSK. It comprises of a number of clinical subtypes, which can be detected and separated into distinct clinical subtypes based on antibody profiling and clinical presentation. Hence, in all patients with myasthenia, it is imperative to look for sources other than AChR by step-wise approach to investigation and most importantly looking for antibodies using antibody profiling.

TAKE HOME MESSAGES

- Autoimmune disorders of the NMJ represent a wide variety of conditions not limited just to presynaptic and postsynaptic disorders
- Agrin, LRP4, MuSK, DOK7, Rapsyn, RyR, titin and voltage-gated potassium channel Kv1.4 are all potential targets of autoimmune attack
- In patients with both AChR and MuSK negative, the possibility of double-seronegative, low affinity AChR antibodies should be looked for
- A combination of fatiguable weakness, myositis, muscle pain and elevated muscle enzymes should raise the suspicion of presence of titin antibodies

- A combination of fatiguable weakness and cardiac problems like myocarditis and arrythmias should raise the suspicion of ryanodine receptor antibodies
- In all patients with NMJ disorders, it is imperative to look for other targets by a stepwise approach to investigations and antibody profiling.

SUGGESTED READINGS

1. Barohn RJ, McIntire D, Herbelin L, et al. Reliability testing of the quantitative myasthenia gravis score. Ann NY Acad Sci. 1998;841:769-72.
2. Carr AS, Cardwell CR, McCarron PO, et al. A systematic review of population based epidemiological studies in myasthenia gravis. BMC Neurol. 2010;10:46.
3. Cortés-Vicente E, Gallardo E, Martínez MÁ, et al. Clinical characteristics of patients with double-seronegative myasthenia gravis and antibodies to cortactin. JAMA Neurol. 2016;73(9):1099-1104.
4. Elmquist D, Lambert EH. Detailed analysis of neuromuscular transmission in a patient with myasthenic syndrome sometimes associated with bronchogenic carcinoma. Mayo Clin Proc. 1968;43:689.
5. Jaretzki A 3rd, Barohn RJ, Ernstoff RM, et al. Myasthenia gravis: Recommendations for clinical research standards. Task Force of the Medical Scientific Advisory Board of the Myasthenia Gravis Foundation of America. Neurology. 2000;55(1):16-23.
6. Koneczny I, Cossins J, Vincent A. The Role of muscle-specific tyrosine kinase (MuSK) and mystery of MuSK myasthenia gravis. J Anat. 2014;224(1):29-35.
7. Lambert EH, Elmqvist D. Quantal components of endplate potentials in myasthenic syndrome. Ann N Y Acad Sci. 1972;183:183-99.
8. Lang B, Newsom Davis J, Wray D, et al. Autoimmune aetiology for myasthenic (Eaton-Lambert) syndrome. Lancet. 1981;2(8240):224-6.
9. Lennon VA, Kryzer TJ, Gnessman GE, et al. Calcium channel antibodies in Lambert–Eaton syndrome and other paraneoplastic syndromes. N Engl J Med. 1995;332:1467-74.
10. Meriggioli MN, Sanders DB. Muscle autoantibodies in myasthenia gravis: Beyond diagnosis? Expert Rev Clin Immunol. 2012;8:427e38.
11. Motomura M, Lang BJ, Vincent A, et al. An improved diagnostic assay for Lambert-Eaton myasthenic syndrome. J Neurol Neurosurg Psychiatry. 1995;58:85-7.
12. Mygland A, Tysnes OB, Aarli JA, et al. IgG subclass distribution of ryanodine receptor autoantibodies in patients with myasthenia gravis and thymoma. J Autoimmun. 1993;6(4):507-15.
13. Nagia L, Lemos J, Abusamra K, et al. Prognosis of ocular myasthenia gravis: Retrospective multicenter analysis. Ophthalmology. 2015;122(7):1517-21.
14. Oh SJ, Kim DE, Kuruoglu R, et al. Diagnostic sensitivity of the laboratory tests in myasthenia gravis. Muscle Nerve. 1992;15(6):720-4.
15. Pascuzzi RM. The edrophonium test. Semin Neurol. 2003;23(1):83-8.
16. Romi F, Suzuki S, Suzuki N, et al. Anti-voltage-gated potassium channel Kv1.4 antibodies in myasthenia gravis. J Neurol. 2011;259(7):1312-6.
17. Sanders DB, Wolfe GI, Benatar M, et al. International consensus guidance for management of myasthenia gravis: Executive summary. Neurology. 2016;87(4):419-25.
18. Skeie GO, Mygland A, Aarli JA, et al. Titin antibodies in patients with late onset myasthenia gravis: Clinical correlations. Autoimmunity. 1995;20(2):99-104.
19. Titulaer MJ, Klooster R, Potman M, et al. SOX antibodies in small-cell lung cancer and Lambert-Eaton myasthenic syndrome: Frequency and relation with survival. J Clin Oncol. 2009;27(26):4260-7.
20. Wang K, McClure J, Tu A. Titin: Major myofibrillar components of striated muscle. Proc Natl Acad Sci USA. 1979;76(8):3698-3702.
21. Yamamoto AM, Gajdos P, Eymard B, et al. Anti-titin antibodies in myasthenia gravis: Tight association with thymoma and heterogeneity of nonthymoma patients. Arch Neurol. 2001;58(6):885-90.
22. Zisimopoulou P, Evangelakou P, Tzartos J, et al. A comprehensive analysis of the epidemiology and clinical characteristics of anti-LRP4 in myasthenia gravis. J Autoimmun. 2014;52:139-45.

CHAPTER 12

Autoimmune Myopathy

Mugundhan Krishnan, Lakshmi Narasimhan Ranganathan, Jawahar Marimuthu, Krishnaprasad TP, Saranya Masilamani, Namrata Jayaharan

INTRODUCTION

Autoimmune myopathies are a heterogenous group of acquired muscle disorders. It is twice more common in women than men. This group of disorders is very rare with an estimated incidence of 4 cases per 100,000 person-years and prevalence of 15–32 cases per 100,000. The hallmark finding is the presence of inflammatory infiltrates on muscle biopsy. The recent identification of antibodies associated with specific myopathies has played an important role in characterizing this disorder. Around 60% of patients with autoimmune myopathy have myositis specific autoantibodies and it is assumed that this frequency may increase when appropriate diagnostic immunoassays are more widely used. The common autoimmune myopathies include dermatomyositis, immune mediated necrotising myopathy, polymyositis, and other overlap syndromes. Inclusion body myositis is also a disorder considered by some authors to be a member of this group of diseases but available pathological evidence suggests that it might actually be a myodegenerative disease associated with accumulation of abnormal proteins.

DERMATOMYOSITIS

Patients with dermatomyositis usually present with both skin and muscle involvement. Even though thought to be a single disease, recent evidence suggests that it may include distinct subtypes associated with unique antibody.

Clinical Features

It has a subacute onset and causes progressive proximal muscle weakness. Patient has difficulty getting up from sitting position and raising arms above shoulders. Patients with severe disease may also present with neck muscle weakness, difficulty swallowing due to pharyngeal weakness, and breathlessness due to diaphragmatic weakness. The weakness is usually painless but may occasionally be associated with myalgia.

Characteristic dermatologic features usually accompany muscle weakness. The rash precedes or occurs at the same time as the weakness. These include Gottron's papules which are scaly erythematous lesions on the extensor surface of metacarpophalangeal joints, and heliotrope rash which are violaceous eruptions on the upper eyelids, occasionally associated with periorbital edema. Both are characteristic of dermatomyositis. Other types of skin manifestations which are less specific are shawl sign, erythematous rash covering the upper arms and shoulders, or a v-shaped rash affecting sun exposed areas on chest. Progressive deposition of calcium as subcutaneous nodules known as calcinosis cutis occurs in some patients.

Interstitial lung disease is present in approximately 20-30% of patients with dermatomyositis and less often joints and cardiac muscle can also be affected. Dermatomyositis is often associated with increased risk of malignancy. Adenocarcinoma is usually detected within 2 years either before or after the development of clinical manifestation of dermatomyositis.

Pathogenesis

Interferon alpha (INF-α) plays an important role in the pathogenesis suggested by the abundance of INF-α in the plasmacytoid dendritic cells infiltrates and the expression levels of INF inducible transcripts in peripheral blood are correlated with disease activity. However, it is unclear how INF-α causes such classic histologic features with perifascicular atrophy.

Antibodies in Dermatomyositis

Myositis specific autoantibodies are present in approximately 60-70% of patients with dermatomyositis and have distinct clinical features. The most common antibody identified in dermatomyositis is autoantibodies recognizing transcriptional intermediary factor 1Y. They are prevalent in nearly 15-40% of dermatomyositis patients. These patients have severe skin manifestations and are at increased risk of cancer.

Antinuclear matrix protein 2 autoantibodies are identified in 40% of dermatomyositis patients and is associated with calcinosis, which is refractory to treatment. Anti-Mi-2 autoantibody is identified in 15% of the patients who present with severe skin manifestation which responds to steroid treatment. Antimelanoma differentiation-associated protein 5 antibody is identified in 5% of patients who have typical skin manifestation of tender palmar papules and have a rapidly progressive interstitial lung disease. Small ubiquitin like modifier 1 autoantibody is present in 8% of the dermatomyositis patients. These patients have skin manifestations before muscle involvement and have associated interstitial lung disease.

Diagnosis

Blood Investigations

Elevated levels of muscle enzymes such as creatine kinase (CK), aldolase, aspartate, and alanine transaminase are present in 90% of the patients. Elevated CK levels are considered more sensitive and specific for muscle damage. However, some patients with classical clinical features may have no CK elevation.

Imaging

Magnetic resonance imaging (MRI) short-TI inversion recovery sequence reveals hyperintense regions corresponding to areas of muscle inflammation or necrosis. Biopsy of the muscles with MRI signal abnormality can increase the diagnostic yield. The T1W images demonstrate muscle replacement by fat and fibrotic tissues.

Electromyography

Typical electromyography findings include small, polyphasic motor units with early recruitment, consistent with myopathic process. Untreated patients have fibrillation potentials and positive sharp waves. The spontaneous activity decreases with steroid treatment.

Histopathology

The hallmark feature of dermatomyositis is perifascicular atrophy where small atrophic fibers line the edges of fascicles that are otherwise composed of relatively normal sized muscle fibers. Perifascicular inflammation with cellular infiltrates composed of macrophages, B-cells and plasmacytoid dendritic cells is a more common but nonspecific finding seen in dermatomyositis. Other less common finding include increased numbers of cytochrome oxidase-deficient fibers suggestive of mitochondrial dysfunction.

NECROTISING AUTOIMMUNE MYOPATHY

Necrotising autoimmune myopthy (NAM) is a subtype of immune mediated myopathies. It is characterized by subacute onset proximal myopathy with elevated CK and biopsy evidence of necrotic myofibres with minimal inflammation.

Pathophysiology

The pathogenesis underlying the initiation of immune process is not clearly understood. However, several studies have stated that genetic susceptibility and statin exposure has led to increased 3-hydroxy-3-methylglutaryl-coenzyme A (HMG-CoA) reductase expression. This over expression further leads to altered processing of HMG-CoA reductase and loss of tolerance to the enzyme leading on to production of autoantibodies against the enzyme. Anti-HMG-CoA reductase autoantibodies recognize the surface antigen on the muscles cells and lead to complement-mediated myonecrosis. This cycle becomes a vicious process even after statin discontinuation as the regenerating muscle fibers serve as sources of autoantigen. The antibody titer correlate with disease severity. Anti-HMG-CoA reductase antibody ELISA (enzyme linked immunosorbent assay) has a sensitivity of 94.4% and specificity of 99.3%.

Anti-HMG-CoA reductase antibody associated myopathy has been found to be strongly associated with HLA-DRB11*01 found in Japanese population. In these genetically susceptible individuals, the presentation of HMG-CoA reductase derived peptides to the immune system leads to the autoimmunity.

Ohnuki et al. found relation between HLADRB1*0803 and anti-signal recognition particle (SRP) in necrotizing autoimmune myopathy. Anti-SRP antibodies are found positive in systemic sclerosis and antisynthetase syndrome.

Less commonly, NAM is found in association with connective tissue disorders like systemic lupus erythematosus (SLE), Sjögren's disease, and scleroderma. A large cohort study by Allenbach et al. found increased association of malignancy in patients diagnosed with NAM and anti-HMG-CoA reductase antibody within a span of 3 years. Around 10% of NAM cases are paraneoplastic. Few case reports shows association of NAM with human immunodeficiency virus and hepatitis C virus.

Clinical Presentation
Subacute progressive proximal myopathy involving the shoulder and pelvic girdle.

Clinical Criteria from the 119th European Neuromuscular Centre International Workshop on Idiopathic Inflammatory Myopathies
- Insidious or subacute onset of proximal muscle weakness with neck flexor involvement
- Elevated CK level
- No ocular weakness
- May be associated with dysphagia, dyspnea, and myalgia
- Exclusion of toxic myopathies, thyroid disease, and muscular dystrophies
- Not associated with rashes and photosensitivity
- Interstitial lung disease and cardiac involvement are reported
- Abnormal electromyography couples with biopsy features suggestive of NAM.

OVERLAP MYOSITIS

When a patient satisfies more than one classification criteria, he is said to have an overlap syndrome. Overlap myositis is the most common inflammatory myopathy according to a study in French Canadian population. It is associated with systemic sclerosis, Sjögren's syndrome, SLE, transfer ribonucleic acid (tRNA) synthetase syndromes, and rheumatoid arthritis, of which association with systemic sclerosis is most common, occurring in around 30% of patients. Myositis is associated with SLE in about 4–16 % of patients.

When a patient presents with features of myositis like proximal muscle weakness, dysphagia, and other confirmatory laboratory investigations, overlap features should be looked for. These include Raynaud's phenomenon, arthritis, scleroderma, sclerodactyly, mechanic's hands, bilateral carpel tunnel syndrome, SLE manifestations, small bowel abnormalities like hypomotility, and malabsorption. If these are present along with the proximal muscle weakness, a diagnosis of overlap myositis is made. Overlap antibodies have further added to the diagnostic accuracy.

Anti-Jo-1 is the most common autoantibody (histidyl tRNA synthetases). Other autoantibodies to tRNA synthetases include EJ, PL-7, PL-12, and KS. These are now included as antisynthetase syndromes. Anti-U1-RNP, anti-U3-RNP, anti-U5-RNP, anti-Ku, and anti-PM/Scl are overlap antibodies associated with systemic sclerosis. Other overlap antibodies include antinucleoporins and anti-SRP.

In a patient with suspected myositis, look for:
- Skeletal muscle involvement
    - Proximal weakness
    - Dysphagia
    - Increased CK
    - Electromyography–myopathic pattern
    - Positive Muscle biopsy
    - Dermatomyositis rash.
- Overlap features
    - Arthritis
    - Mechanic's hands
    - Scleroderma
    - Sclerodactyly

    - Carpel tunnel syndrome
    - Systemic lupus erythematosus manifestations.
- Overlap autoantibodies
    - Antisynthetases
    - Scleroderma associated autoantibodies
    - Anti-SRP
    - Antinucleoporin.

Then classify the myositis:
- Overlap features + autoantibodies—overlap myositis
- Characteristic rash and antibody of dermatomyositis—dermatomyositis
- Lack of clinical and serological correlates—polymyositis.

Overlap myositis and polymyositis have a low risk for cancer in contrast to dermatomyositis.

The autoantibodies help predict the course of arthritis, which may be monophasic or chronic which aids in planning the management.

Overlap antibodies to U1-RNP, PM/Scl, and Ku have a monophasic course and respond to initial treatment with steroids. Antibodies to nucleoporins, SRP, and synthetases have a chronic course and require immunosuppressive agents in addition to steroids.

ANTISYNTHETASE SYNDROME

Myositis associated with aminoacyl tRNA synthetase is found in 20% of cases and is called antisynthetase syndrome. The most common among them is antihistidyl-tRNA synthetase (anti Jo-1). It is a multisystem disease which requires two or more of the following–myositis, arthritis, Raynaud's phenomenon, fever, interstitial lung disease, and mechanic's hand. It may be associated with a rash causing confusion with dermatomyositis, but the biopsy findings are different.

Patients with anti-Jo-1 antibodies have perifascicular necrosis with sarcolemmal deposition of complement which is different from the perifascicular atrophy seen in patients with dermatomyositis.

INCLUSION BODY MYOSITIS

In addition to dermatomyositis, immune necrotizing myopathy, and polymyositis, inclusion body myositis (IBM) has also been included in this category. It has characteristic clinical and pathological features and a poor response to treatment.

Of the immune mediated disorders, IBM is associated with maximum inflammation. The inflammatory infiltrate consists of B-cells, plasma cells, macrophages, dendritic cells, and cytotoxic T-cells. There is a link between IBM and T-cell granular lymphocytic leukemia.

The median age of onset is after 40 years. It characteristically involves quadriceps (vastus medialis and lateralis > rectus femoris), finger flexors, and ankle dorsiflexors. The involvement is focal and asymmetric. Other muscles like biceps brachii, wrist flexors, and triceps are also involved. Facial involvement is common. Simple physical examination identifying distal muscle involvement helps in earlier diagnosis.

Diagnosis

- Creatine kinase is elevated, 5–10 times the upper limit of normal. More than a 10-fold elevation excludes the diagnosis

- Electromyography shows fibrillation, sharp positive waves, and occasional large motor units which lead to confusion with amyotrophic lateral sclerosis
- Magnetic resonance imaging shows patchy areas of muscle involvement and replacement with fatty tissue
- Biomarkers: A significant improvement is the identification of the autoantigen NT5C1A and its autoantibody which has a specificity of 87–100%
- Muscle biopsy shows both inflammatory and degenerative changes. Inflammatory changes show endomysial inflammation with non-necrotic muscle fibers surrounded and invaded by lymphocytes. The lymphocytes cause nodular infiltrates and cause displacement of myofibrils. Degenerative changes are postulated to be secondary to autoimmunity due to the presence of NT5C1A around the rimmed vacuoles. The changes include rimmed vacuoles, tubulofilaments, and cytomembranous whorls.

POLYMYOSITIS

With the recognition of autoantibodies and characteristic biopsy features, polymyositis has become a rare diagnosis among patients with autoimmune myopathy. The earlier criteria for polymyositis included symmetric proximal muscle weakness, absence of dermatomyositis rash, elevated muscle enzymes, electromyography showing myopathic pattern, muscle biopsy showing inflammation, or necrosis. An important inclusion criteria is the presence of non-necrotic muscle cells surrounded or invaded by lymphocytes and exclusion criteria is the presence of muscle weakness characteristic of IBM. No polymyositis specific autoantibodies have been identified so far. Prior to the recognition of anti-SRP, anti-HMG-CoA reductase, and anti-NT5C1A, autoimmune necrotizing myopathy and IBM would have been classified as polymyositis. Presence of perifascicular atrophy with or without the rash is suggestive of dermatomyositis. Even limb girdle muscular dystrophy was classified as polymyositis due to the presence of an inflammatory infiltrate. Thus, the presence of biomarkers and characteristic biopsy features have made polymyositis a diagnosis of exclusion.

TREATMENT

There is no class 1 recommendations for specific therapy in autoimmune myopathy. Initial therapy in these patients include oral prednisone at a dose of 1 mg/kg/day. In severely affected patients, oral course is preceded by 3 days of intravenous methyl prednisolone therapy.

With side effects of long-term steroids, patients can be started on steroid sparing agents like methotrexate, azathioprine, and mycophenolate mofetil. Azathioprine is preferred in patients with interstitial lung disease. In those patients with very severe weakness or who do not respond to initial combination of medications after 6-8 weeks, intravenous immunoglobulins or rituximab can be tried. Rituximab is more responsive in patients with refractory anti-SRP positive NAM.

Once muscle strength returns to normal or have reached the plateau phase, steroids are slowly tapered by reducing 10 mg/day every 3-4 weeks. After reaching 20 mg/day, further reduction of 5 mg/day every 4 weeks is made. At the start of first sign of disease flare up, more aggressive treatment has to be restarted. Careful monitoring of muscle strength and serum CK levels during the course of tapering is required. Few cases show persisting muscle weakness in the context of normal CK levels which signifies severe myopathic state characterized by fatty replacement of myofibres and thereby no muscle necrosis to cause enzyme elevation. This is often seen in patients with dermatomyositis.

In patients who have no evidence of active disease for 6–12 months after withdrawal of steroids, other therapeutic agents in use could also be tapered and discontinued.

Patients with anti-HMG-CoA reductase and anti-SRP positive NAM require multiple agents particularly in statin-naive cases.

CONCLUSION

Autoimmune myopathies like dermatomyositis, immune necrotizing myopathy, and overlap myositis have unique clinical and pathological characteristics with myositis associated antibodies. Overlap myositis should always be considered and features of connective tissue disease should be actively looked for. Inclusion body myositis should be suspected with the characteristic pattern of muscle involvement. As mentioned earlier, polymyositis is now a diagnosis of exclusion. All these disorders are treated with nonspecific immunosuppressive medication. With advances in the mechanisms of pathogenesis, more specific treatment will be developed in the future.

TAKE HOME MESSAGES

- Autoimmune myopathy is a treatable myopathy which has to be diagnosed and treated appropriately
- Specific autoantibodies are associated with unique clinical phenotypes and may be used for diagnostic and prognostic purposes
- Neuronal antibody evaluation is an important tool in diagnosis of suspected autoimmune neurological syndromes
- History and family history of autoimmune disease, history and family history of cancer, and clinical signs suggestive of autoimmunity on examination are the clues for initiating neuronal antibody evaluation.

SUGGESTED READINGS

1. András C, Ponyi A, Constantin T, et al. Dermatomyositis and polymyositis associated with malignancy: A 21-year retrospective study. J Rheumatol. 2008;35(3)438Y444.
2. Allenbach Y, Keraen J, Bouvier AM, et al. High risk of cancer in autoimmune necrotizing myopathies: usefulness of myositis specific antibody. Brain. 2016;139(8):2131-5.
3. Greenberg SA. Inclusion body myositis. Continuum (Minneap Minn). 2016;22(6, Muscle and Neuromuscular Junction Disorders):1871-88.
4. Greenberg SA. Theories of the pathogenesis of inclusion body myositis. Curr Rheumatol Rep. 2010;12:221-8.
5. Karpati G, O'Ferrall EK. Sporadic inclusion body myositis:pathogenic considerations. Ann Neurol. 2009;65:7-11.
6. Mammen AL. Autoimmune myopathies. Continuum (Minneap Minn). 2016;22(6, Muscle and Neuromuscular Junction Disorders):1852-70.
7. Mammen AL. Autoimmune myopathies: Autoantibodies, phenotypes and pathogenesis. Nat Rev Neurol. 2011;7(6):343-54.
8. Ohnuki Y, Suzuki S, Shiina T, et al. HLA-DRB1 alleles in immune-mediated necrotizing myopathy. Neurology. 2016:10-212.
9. Siegal FP, Kadowaki N, Shodell M, et al. The nature of the principal type 1 interferonproducing cells in human blood. Science. 1999;284(5421);1835-7.

10. Smoyer-Tomic KE, Amato AA, Fernandes AW. Incidence and prevalence of idiopathic inflammatory myopathies among commercially insured, medicare supplemental insured, and medicaid enrolled populations: An administrative claims analysis. 2012;13:103.
11. Troyanav Y, Targoff IN, Payette MP, et al. Redefining dermatomyositis: A description of new diagnostic criteria that differentiate pure dermatomyositis from overlap myositis with dermatomyositis features. Medicine (Baltimore). BMC Musculoskelet Disord. 2014;93(24):414.
12. Walsh RJ, Kong SW, Yao Y, et al. Type I interferon-inducible gene expression in blood is present and reflects disease activity in dermatomyositis and polymyositis. Arthritis Rheum. 2007;56(11): 3784-92.

Immunotherapy

Sruthi S Nair, Soumya Sundaram, Muralidharan Nair

INTRODUCTION

Autoimmune neurological diseases are a heterogeneous group of conditions with highly variable clinical presentations. Distinguishing these conditions from the degenerative and structural diseases is cardinal as they are amenable to treatment on the one hand and pose risk of relapses and continued disease activity with inadequate treatment on the other. The repertoire of drugs used for treatment of these disorders is ever expanding with newer molecules being added every year.

IMMUNOMODULATORY THERAPY

The drugs which act by modifying the immune mechanisms of the body are called immunomodulators. Most of these drugs are immunosuppressants and selectively or nonselectively suppress the effector cells of the immune system. Box 1 lists the medications and procedures used in immunotherapy of neurological disorders.

The therapy in autoimmune disorders involves two phases—(1) the treatment of acute disease or relapse, and (2) long-term maintenance immunotherapy. The acute treatment is aimed at terminating the inflammation and/or removal of the pathogenic antibodies. High dose corticosteroids, intravenous immunoglobulin (IVIG) and plasma exchange (PE) form the mainstay of acute therapy. All chronic or relapsing disorders need treatment with a maintenance immunotherapy which is generally achieved with the use of oral steroids, cytotoxic therapy, and monoclonal antibodies (mAb). In relapsing forms of multiple sclerosis (MS), a plethora of drugs are available for control of disease activity and relapse prevention.

The modalities of immunotherapy are discussed in detail in this chapter.

GLUCOCORTICOIDS

Corticosteroids have been in clinical use since 1929 and continue to be the most extensively used immunomodulatory agents, with efficacy demonstrated in a wide range of neurological conditions. They are beneficial both in acute situations and for long-term immunomodulation, although most of the data derives from case series and clinical experience rather than randomized trials.

The wide range of activity of the steroids is related to the ubiquitous presence of their receptors throughout the body, in particular, the lymphoid system. Steroids induce redistribution of lymphocytes resulting in peripheral lymphopenia. They act

> **Box 1: Immunotherapeutic drugs in neurology**
> - Acute/maintenance therapy
>   - Glucocorticoids
>   - Intravenous immunoglobulin
>   - Therapeutic plasma exchange
> - Maintenance therapy
>   - Antimetabolites or antiproliferative agents
>   - Azathioprene
>   - Mycophenolate mofetil
>   - Methotrexate
>   - Cyclophosphamide
>   - Mitoxantrone
>   - Teriflunomide
>   - Calcineurin inhibitors
>   - Cyclosporine
>   - Tacrolimus
>   - Monoclonal antibodies
>   - Rituximab
>   - Natalizumab
>   - Daclizumab
>   - Alemtuzumab
>   - Ocrelizumab
>   - Recombinant cytokines
>   - Interferon beta-1a
>   - Interferon beta-1b
>   - Synthetic polypeptide
>   - Glatiramer acetate
>   - Sphingosine 1-phosphate modulator
>   - Fingolimod
>   - Nrf2 [nuclear factor (erythroid-derived 2)-like 2] activators
>   - Dimethyl fumarate
>   - Miscellaneous drugs
>   - Isoprinosine
>   - Levamisole
>   - Thalidomide
> - Autologous hematopoietic stem cell transplantation

on intracellular receptors to regulate gene transcription, produce downregulation of proinflammatory cytokines, inhibit T-cell proliferation and antigen presentation and reduce chemotaxis of neutrophils and monocytes.

The common steroids administered parenterally are methyl prednisolone and dexamethasone and the best-studied oral steroids are prednisolone and dexamethasone. The different strategies of steroid administration in common autoimmune disorders are outlined in Table 1.

Long-term use of steroids is associated with significant multisystemic side effects. They include weight gain, Cushingoid facies (moon face with plethoric cheeks), redistribution of fat (buffalo hump, increased abdominal fat), hyperglycemia, hypertension, increased appetite, obesity, avascular necrosis of femoral head, osteoporosis, myopathy, increased susceptibility to infections, thinning of skin, easy bruisability, and poor wound healing.

Intermittent pulse steroid therapy (administration of suprapharmacological doses over a short period) for maintenance is suggested as an option to reduce the long-term toxicity, but needs validation in neurological diseases.

PLASMA EXCHANGE

The word "apheresis" is derived from Greek and literally means "to separate" or "to remove". This term refers to the various processes by which blood is separated into its components.

Immunotherapy

TABLE 1: Strategies for steroid treatment in common neuroimmunological diseases

Short course therapy	
500–1,000 mg (or 30 mg/kg if weight <30 kg) methyl prednisolone intravenous for 3–5 days with fast taper	
Acute attack or relapse of multiple sclerosis	Oral prednisolone tapering may or may not be given over 1–3 weeks
Acute disseminated encephalomyelitis	Oral prednisolone to be started at 1 mg/kg/day and then to be tapered over 4–6 weeks
Pulse therapy with prolonged tapering	
1,000 mg methyl prednisolone intravenous for 5 days followed by oral prednisolone 1 mg/kg tapered slowly	
Neuromyelitis optica with relapse	Needs steroid sparing agent to be started, prednisolone to be tapered once alternate agent becomes active
N-methyl-D-aspartate receptor encephalitis	Usually pulse steroid is concurrently given with other acute therapy, oral prednisolone tapered over many weeks, immunosuppression with steroid-sparing agent at least for 1 year
High dose oral therapy, pulse therapy in severe cases	
Oral prednisolone at 0.75–1.5 mg/kg/day till disease remission and then slowly tapered over many months with or without steroid-sparing agents.	
In severe presentations, 1,000 mg methyl prednisolone intravenous for 3–5 days can be given	
Neurosarcoidosis	Tapering dose steroid therapy at least for 6–12 months, usually has steroid dependence
Polymyositis and dermatomyositis	Steroid taper after weakness or creatine kinase normalizes or stabilizes (usually 3–6 months)
Oral therapy alone	
Oral prednisolone at 1–1.5 mg/kg/day till remission and then slow taper	
Chronic inflammatory demyelinating polyradiculoneuropathy	Steroid-sparing therapy in case of side effects or inadequate response
Myasthenia gravis	High dose strategy can sometimes produce transient worsening and crisis, hence slow escalation starting from 5 mg/day to 10 mg/day of prednisolone is preferred

The most common therapeutic procedure performed with apheresis is the therapeutic PE. This involves the removal of a large volume of plasma with substitution of the volume with replacement fluids. This should be differentiated from the term "plasmapheresis" which implies the removal of the plasma component of blood without replacement of the fluid and can hence be performed only in small volumes.

Venous access can be obtained with a central or peripheral catheter. Therapeutic PE can be performed by membrane filtration (which separates components by size) or by continuous or discontinuous centrifugation (which separates components by density). The plasma component is removed and cells are mixed with replacement fluid before returning to the patient. The preferred replacement fluid for maintenance of intravascular volume is albumin diluted in saline; however, the cost is limiting. If plasma is used as replacement, it should be reserved for the later stages of the procedure.

Plasma exchange is used most commonly as an acute therapy in immune-mediated disorders. The mechanism in autoimmune disorders is thought to be removal of pathogenic antibodies, immune complexes, and cytokines. However, an immunomodulatory mechanism is also postulated in view of the prolonged response after PE. This could be mediated by an anti-inflammatory shift of the T helper cell population and suppression of interferon (IFN)-gamma and interleukin (IL)-2 production induced by PE.

About 60–70% of the pathogenic substances are removed for every 1–1.5 plasma volume (40–50 mL/kg body weight per exchange) exchanged. Patients with neurological disease usually have five exchanges daily or alternate days, which can reduce the immunoglobulin (Ig) levels by more than 90%. The therapeutic indications for PE are given in Table 2.

TABLE 2: Therapeutic indications for plasma exchange and intravenous immunoglobulin

Level of evidence	Plasma exchange	Intravenous immunoglobulin
Level A (Established effective)	• Severe GBS • CIDP, short-term treatment	• GBS in adults • Long-term treatment of CIDP • Stiff person syndrome • Acute multiple sclerosis if other drugs not tolerated or in pregnancy/postpartum
Level B (Probably effective)	• Polyneuropathy with IgA or IgG monoclonal gammopathy • Mild GBS • Steroid-resistant exacerbations in relapsing multiple sclerosis	• Moderate to severe myasthenia gravis • Multifocal motor neuropathy
Level C (Possibly effective)	Fulminant demyelinating CNS disease	• Nonresponsive dermatomyositis in adults • Necrotizing autoimmune myopathy • Lambert–Eaton myasthenic syndrome • Acute disseminated encephalomyelitis
Level U (insufficient evidence)	• Myasthenia gravis—crisis and preoperative preparation • (PANDAS) • Sydenham chorea	• Neuromyelitis optica • Autoimmune epilepsy • Polymyositis • IgM paraprotein associated neuropathy • Diabetic radiculoplexoneuropathy Miller Fisher syndrome • Children with GBS • Vasculitic neuropathy
Ineffective	• Chronic or secondary progressive multiple sclerosis • Polyneuropathy with IgM monoclonal gammopathy of undetermined significance	• Inclusion body myositis • Postpolio syndrome

CIDP, chronic inflammatory demyelinating polyradiculoneuropathy; CNS, central nervous system; GBS, Guillain-Barre syndrome; IgA, immunoglobulin A; IgG, immunoglobulin G; PANDAS, pediatric autoimmune neuropsychiatric disorders associated with streptococcal infections.

The effects of PE are usually rapid and temporary. Resynthesis and redistribution of plasma proteins between intra and extravascular space cause reaccumulation of the plasma proteins removed by PE. Immunoglobulin, especially IgG, has a low turnover rate and may remain low in plasma for up to 5 weeks after PE. Benefits are the highest when used for self-limiting diseases like Guillain–Barre syndrome (GBS) and when a rapid therapeutic action is desired as in myasthenic crisis. It has far less use as a chronic maintenance therapy, partly due to the difficulty in obtaining venous access.

Plasma exchange is associated with many complications with rates ranging from 5% to 36%. These complications may result from the procedure itself or due to the catheter used for intravenous access. The common local reactions are local paresthesias, urticaria, bleeding and hematoma and systemic reactions including vasovagal reaction, hypotension, nausea and vomiting. Hypotension is a major limiting side effect and should be watched for and prevented by avoiding antihypertensives and adequately hydrating patients before and during the procedure. Catheter-related side effects are common and include catheter block, thrombosis or hematoma, and catheter related sepsis and infections. Plasma exchange can also alter the blood levels of drugs, especially IVIG.

INTRAVENOUS IMMUNOGLOBULIN

Intravenous immunoglobulin is pooled human IgG which is made safe for infusion in humans. The discovery of its efficacy in autoimmune disorders was made serendipitously in 1981, when IVIG therapy in children with coexisting hypogammaglobulinemia and idiopathic thrombocytopenic purpura was observed to produce improvement in platelet count. This led way to the use of IVIG in several other diseases with a confirmed or suspected autoimmune etiology.

Commercially available IVIG is produced by cold ethanol fractionation of human plasma derived from pools of 3,000–10,000 donors to precipitate the IgG fraction. The final product contains more than 95% IgG and around 2.5% IgA. The large pool of donors accounts for the diversity of antibodies which is essential for the biological action of the agent.

Intravenous immunoglobulin has actions at multiple levels and pinpointing the exact therapeutic mechanism is difficult. The most plausible mechanism is the presence of anti-idiotypic antibodies within the IVIG which bind to the variable region or idiotype of the pathogenic antibodies and then regulate and suppress their production. Other mechanisms include inhibition of complement pathway and formation of membrane attack complex, downregulation of Ig production from T-cells, saturation of Fc receptors on macrophages and other effector cells, enhancement of suppressor T-cell activity, suppression of pathogenic cytokines like IL-1, tumor necrosis factor (TNF)-α, and IL-1β, neutralization of viruses inducing autoimmune disease, effects on cell migration by modulation of adhesion molecules and inhibition of lymphocyte proliferation and effect on remyelination.

The commonly used dosage is 2 g/kg body weight over 5 days, with infusion rate not exceeding 200 mL/hour. Clinical indications are detailed in Table 2. Most of the adverse effects are minor. Infusion related complications occur in less than 10% of patients and are related to the presence of Ig aggregates in the infusion. Life threatening anaphylaxis occurs very rarely, especially in those with IgA deficiency and common variable immunodeficiency who have antibodies to IgA. Determination of serum IgA levels prior to infusion may be done to avoid this.

Intravenous immunoglobulin can induce increase in serum viscosity and thromboembolic events. Headache and aseptic meningitis can occur and usually subside in 24–48 hours with analgesics. Skin reactions and very rarely renal tubular necrosis can occur which are reversible. Serological tests, erythrocyte sedimentation rate and serum sodium levels are influenced by infusion and the false results may persist up to 1 month.

Compared to PE, IVIG has many advantages. It does not remove plasma proteins, is useful in patients with nutritional deficiency, there is no risk of hypovolemia (useful in autonomic instability and cardiac disease), is less immunosuppressive, does not alter the serum drug levels and is easy to administer. The effectiveness of IVIG is not restricted to antibody-mediated disorders. The major drawbacks are the temporary effects (half-life 18–32 days) and the prohibitive cost.

CYTOTOXIC THERAPIES

Long-term maintenance in many of the autoimmune disorders requires the use of steroid-sparing agents. The most commonly used drugs are antimetabolites (which interfere with synthesis of DNA). They are nonselective immunosuppressants and prone to long-term toxicity, but are preferred in many instances due to the long-term clinical experience with these drugs. Most of these drugs produce optimal clinical effectiveness after a few months of initiation so that alternate immunotherapy is required during this period. Tables 3 and 4 summarize the mechanisms, adverse effects and clinical applications of these agents.

Azathioprine

The active metabolite of azathioprine (AZA) is 6-mercaptopurine (6-MP) which is further broken down to inactive metabolites by thiopurine S-methyltransferase (TPMT) and xanthine oxidase. The active metabolite 6-MP interferes with purine nucleotide synthesis, thus inhibiting lymphocyte proliferation. Azathioprine is extensively used as an immunosuppressive agent in the demyelinating disorders, autoimmune encephalitis and immune-mediated neuromuscular disorders. It is started at a low dose of 25 mg and slowly titrated to the optimal dosage depending on the blood count and liver enzymes. Lymphocyte count between 600/µL and 1,000/µL and an increase of mean erythrocyte corpuscular volume by 5% from baseline is optimal for patients on AZA therapy. The effect of this drug is seen after long-term use usually after 1 year. The major side effects include recurrent infections, leukopenia, thrombocytopenia and hepatic dysfunction. Frequent monitoring of blood counts including platelet count and liver functions is required. The myelosuppressive effects are more prominent in people who have low-intermediate activity of TPMT, a result of genetic polymorphism, and should be considered in patients with cytopenias at low doses of AZA.

Mycophenolate Mofetil

Mycophenolic acid (MPA) is the active metabolite of mycophenolate mofetil (MMF). Mycophenolic acid reversibly inhibits inosine monophosphate dehydrogenase which is involved in guanosine nucleotide synthesis. The immunosuppressive effects are mediated through reduction in T- and B-lymphocytes proliferation, antibody formation and cell-mediated responses. Due to modest side effect profile when compared to other cytotoxic agents, MMF is used in many immune-mediated diseases. The usual dose of MMF is 1–3 g/day with regular monitoring of blood counts with a target absolute lymphocyte count of 1,000–1,500/µL.

TABLE 3: Mechanism of action and adverse effects of common cytotoxic agents

Drug name	Mechanism of action	Immunological effects	Adverse effects
Mitoxantrone	DNA topoisomerase II inhibitor	Inhibits B-cells, T-cells and macrophages, increases suppressor T-cell function, inhibits migration of monocytes and lymphocytes, induces apoptosis of dendritic cells, decreases cytokine levels	Immunosuppression, bone marrow suppression, secondary leukemia, cardiotoxicity, infertility, amenorrhea, alopecia, vomiting
Azathioprine	Purine synthesis inhibitor	Inhibition of lymphocyte proliferation	Leukopenia, thrombocytopenia, hepatitis, pancreatitis, recurrent infections and malignancy
Mycophenolate mofetil	Inhibits inosine monophosphate dehydrogenase	Potent cytostatic effect on lymphocytes, induces T-cell apoptosis, reduces expression of adhesion molecules and thereby recruitment of lymphocytes and monocytes, reduced nitric oxide synthesis	Diarrhea, abdominal pain, leucopenia, drug-induced fever, infections and lymphoma
Methotrexate	Competitive inhibitor of dihydrofolate reductase and thymidylate synthase	Lymphocyte depletion, potentiates anti-inflammatory effects of adenosine, decreases inflammatory cytokines	Hepatic dysfunction, cirrhosis, acute and chronic interstitial pneumonitis, diarrhea, hemorrhagic colitis and intestinal perforation, stomatitis, cytopenias, fatal skin reactions, lymphoma
Cyclosporin	Inhibition of calcineurin/NFAT pathway and blockade of JNK and p38 signaling pathway	Antiproliferative effects on T helper cells, decrease in IL-2 production	Nephrotoxicity, hypertension, neurotoxicity (tremor, confusion), gastrointestinal (abdominal cramps, diarrhea), gum hypertrophy, infections and malignancy (lymphoma)
Cyclophosphamide	Metabolites form cross-links with DNA strands and prevent DNA replication	• Inhibits humoral and cell-mediated immune response, • Selectively targets CD45/CD4+RA+T-cells and increases the number of Th2 cells	Second malignancy (bladder, myeloproliferative and lymphoproliferative), amenorrhea, infertility, hemorrhagic cystitis, infections, cardiotoxicity, cytopenias, alopecia, rare fatal skin reactions

IL, interleukin; JNK, c-Jun N-terminal kinases; NFAT, nuclear factor of activated T-cells.

TABLE 4: Indications, doses and monitoring of cytotoxic agents

Drug	Indications	Dose	Monitor
Mitoxantrone	Secondary progressive, progressive relapsing and aggressive relapsing remitting multiple sclerosis	12 mg/m² per dose as intravenous once in 3 months (maximum cumulative dose of 140 mg/m²)	CBC, LFT, LVEF before each dose and thereafter annually after completion of treatment
Azathioprine	NMOSD, autoimmune encephalitis, myasthenia gravis, CIDP	2–3 mg/kg	CBC, LFT once a week during titration and monthly for next 3 months, followed by once every 3 months
Mycophenolate mofetil	CIDP, MMCB, mononeuritis multiplex, myasthenia gravis, inflammatory myopathy, NMOSD, multiple sclerosis, autoimmune encephalitis	1–3 g/day per oral in 2–3 divided doses	CBC and LFT monthly for initial 6 months and later twice a year
Methotrexate	Myasthenia gravis, inflammatory myopathy, NMOSD, neurosarcoidosis	5 mg/week and slow escalation up to a maximum dose of 20 mg/week	CBC, LFT and RFT every 2 weeks till the optimal dose is reached and thereafter monthly for the next 1 year. Once disease and dose is stable, monitoring is done once in 3 months
Cyclosporin	Myasthenia gravis and multiple sclerosis	2.5 mg/kg/day with slow titration of 0.5 mg/kg/day dose every 4–8 weeks. Maximum dose is 5 mg/kg/day	CBC, RFT, drug level, blood pressure
Cyclophosphamide	CNS vasculitis, vasculitic mononeuritis multiplex, inflammatory myopathy, autoimmune encephalitis	500–750 mg/m2 per dose intravenous every month for 6 months	CBC, RFT, urine routine before each dose

CBC, complete blood count; LFT, liver function test; MMCB, multifocal motor neuropathy with conduction block; NMOSD, neuromyelitis optica spectrum disorder; RFT, renal function test; LVEF, left ventricular ejection fraction; CIPD, Chronic inflammatory demyelinating polyneuropathy; CNS, central nervous system.

Methotrexate

Methotrexate (MTX) is a folate antagonist and it exerts antiproliferative effects on lymphocytes by inhibiting purine and pyrimidine synthesis. In addition, MTX reduces inflammatory cytokine levels and antigen-stimulated T-cell response and potentiates anti-inflammatory action of adenosine by its release. Methotrexate is started at a weekly dose of 7.5–10 mg with slow titration of 2.5–5 mg every month depending on the laboratory parameters. Doses more than 7.5–10 mg/week, has to be administered twice a week for better bioavailability. Concomitant use of folic or folinic acid (not on the same day of MTX dose) to prevent gastrointestinal and hepatic side effects is advised.

Cyclosporine

Cyclosporine (CsA) is a polypeptide immunosuppressive agent and is highly efficacious for prevention of organ transplant rejection. Cyclosporine binds with cyclophilin forming CsA-cyclophilin complex which inhibits calcineurin/nuclear factor of activated T-cells (NFAT) pathway ultimately leading to inhibition of T helper cell proliferation. Cyclosporine is used off-label in refractory cases of MS and myasthenia gravis; however, experience is very limited in these neurological conditions. The major adverse effect related to CsA use is acute and chronic nephrotoxicity. Acute nephrotoxicity is reversible and is due to afferent arteriolar constriction, whereas chronic nephrotoxicity is due to renal fibrosis. Blood concentration of the drug should be regularly monitored in view of the narrow therapeutic range.

Cyclophosphamide

Cyclophosphamide (CYP) is a synthetic antineoplastic drug which is used as second- or third-line agent in many immune-mediated neurological disorders. Cyclophosphamide acts by introducing alkyl radicals into DNA strands forming DNA cross-links, thus interfering with DNA replication. Cyclophosphamide is indicated in central nervous system (CNS) vasculitis, vasculitic mononeuritis multiplex, neuromyelitis optica spectrum disorder (NMOSD), inflammatory myopathy and autoimmune encephalitis. To prevent hemorrhagic cystitis, intravenous or oral 2-mercaptoethanesulfonate sodium (Mesna) and forced diuresis is advised along with CYP.

Mitoxantrone

Mitoxantrone is a synthetic anthracenedione, initially developed as an antineoplastic agent, and is approved for use in secondary progressive, progressive relapsing, and aggressive relapsing remitting MS. It is also used in NMOSD when first- and second-line agents fail. Mitoxantrone intercalates with DNA through hydrogen bonds and causes cross-linking and breakage of DNA strands. It also inhibits topoisomerase II, thus interfering with DNA repair mechanism. It produces global immunosuppression by affecting the proliferation of B-cells, T-cells and macrophages, and also by reducing the inflammatory cytokines (TNF-α, IL and IFN gamma). Patients mandatorily require monitoring for cardiotoxicity (electrocardiogram and echocardiogram) and blood counts prior to each dose and on treatment completion.

INTERFERON

Interferons (IFNs) are a family of naturally occurring cytokines which possess antiviral and antitumor activities and play an important role in regulating the immune response. Therapeutically useful IFNs are pure recombinant forms prepared in culture of which IFNα has potent antineoplastic and antiviral properties and IFNβ has shown efficacy in relapsing remitting multiple sclerosis (RRMS).

Interferon Beta

Therapeutic forms of IFNβ can be produced from eukaryotic cell lines (IFNβ-1a) or from bacterial cell lines (IFNβ-1b). Both have application in the treatment of RRMS. Multiple randomized controlled trials have proven their benefit in reducing the annualized relapse rates by 18–34% with higher efficacy for higher doses.

Interferon beta-1a and -1b have similar mechanisms of action in spite of their structural differences. They bind to type I IFN receptor to produce changes in gene transcription which shifts the immune system from a proinflammatory to an anti-inflammatory state. They impair effector T-cell function at multiple levels, inhibit antigen presentation, downregulate inflammatory cytokines, and augment suppressor T-cells. They also inhibit the expression of major histocompatibility complex class II on endothelial cells contributing to blood–brain barrier, prevent leukocyte adhesion to cerebral endothelium, and induce release of nerve growth factor from astrocytes.

Interferon beta-1b is administered subcutaneously at a dose of 250 μg every alternate day. Interferon beta-1a is available as an intramuscular preparation to be given 30 μg once a week or subcutaneous preparation to be taken 22 μg or 44 μg thrice a week.

Side effects are common but nonhazardous. They include flu-like symptoms (fever, headache, malaise) and injection site reactions, both of which tend to reduce over time. Interferons are immunogenic and can induce the development of neutralizing antibodies which occur persistently in 5–30% of the treated patients and reduce the treatment efficacy. They occur usually in the first year of treatment and more commonly in those receiving IFNβ-1b.

MONOCLONAL ANTIBODIES

Monoclonal antibodies are synthesized by clones of cells formed by the hybridization of B-cells and myeloma cell lines. This fusion produces cells which can produce unlimited quantities of a desired antibody. All the antibodies from a single clone target a single epitope and are, therefore, termed monoclonal.

The terminology of mAbs is derived from the origins of their constant or Fc region which binds to cells and variable region or Fv which interact with unique antigens. The mAbs were traditionally cultured from a foreign host such as mice to which human body mounts an immune response. To avoid these, the cells can be made:
- using transgenic mice which creates antibodies with human Fc regions (suffix—zumab),
- by splitting the host-derived mAb and combining the created Fv region with human Fc region (suffix—ximab), or
- creating a fusion protein composed of human Fc region and an antigen-specific receptor which is different in structure from a classical antibody (suffix—cept).

  In neurology, mAbs have found the greatest application in the treatment of MS.

Natalizumab

Natalizumab is a humanized antibody directed against α4β1 integrin. Natalizumab blocks the adhesion of the activated T lymphocytes to vascular endothelium and prevents their migration across the BBB. The drug is highly efficacious and reduces annualized relapse rate by 63% and occurrence of new gadolinium enhancing lesions by 92%. It is administered monthly at a dose of 300 mg, as intravenous infusion.

The major adverse effect with natalizumab is the risk of progressive multifocal leukoencephalopathy (PML) which is an opportunistic infection caused by the John Cunningham (JC) polyomavirus. There is higher risk of PML in patients with JC virus antibody positivity, longer duration of treatment (more than 2 years) and previous use of immunosuppressive drugs. As a result, the drug is reserved for patients who are nonresponsive to first-line therapies or who have an aggressive disease course.

Rituximab

This chimeric antibody selectively targets CD20 positive B-cells and has demonstrated efficacy in a variety of autoimmune CNS disorders. It depletes peripheral blood B-cells by complement activation and membrane attack complex formation, antibody-dependent cellular cytotoxicity, and induction of apoptosis.

Two schedules of dosing are commonly followed—375 mg/m² weekly for 4 weeks, or two infusions of 1 g, 2 weeks apart. The depletion of B-cells starts 1 month after the administration and reappearance in circulation by 6–8 months. The infusions can be repeated after 6–12 months. Monitoring can be done by measuring quantum of CD19 positive lymphocytes as CD20 positive cells may be reduced by passive blocking.

The adverse effects include infusion-related reactions, hypotension, flu-like symptoms, anaphylactic or skin reactions and the rare, but serious cytokine release syndrome. Reactivation of tuberculosis or hepatitis should be considered and patient should be evaluated thoroughly before starting therapy.

Rituximab has been found effective in a number of neurological conditions. Efficacy in RRMS and anti-myelin associated glycoprotein polyneuropathy is shown in controlled trials while uncontrolled trials claim efficacy in NMOSD, multifocal motor neuropathy, paraneoplastic neurological disorders, autoimmune myopathies and myasthenia gravis.

Other Monoclonal Antibodies

Most of the other mAbs are used in the treatment of RRMS and are detailed in Table 5. Tumor necrosis factor-α blocking agents (infliximab and etanercept) may be beneficial in polymyositis and dermatomyositis.

MISCELLANEOUS IMMUNOMODULATORY THERAPY

A host of oral medications with diverse mechanisms of action have emerged in the management of MS and they are elaborated in Table 5. Autologous hematopoietic stem cell transplantation, which resets the immune system, is also administered in refractory cases of RRMS.

TABLE 5: Drugs approved by regulatory agencies for relapse prevention in multiple sclerosis

Agent	Mechanism of action	Dose and route	Side effects	Remarks
Interferon beta-1a	Reduces BBB disruption and modulates T-cell, B-cell, and cytokine functions	30 μg once a week IM	Flu-like symptoms, injection site reactions, allergy, elevated liver enzymes, depression	18% reduction in ARR
Interferon beta-1a	Reduces BBB disruption and modulates T-cell, B-cell, and cytokine functions	22 μg or 44 μg thrice a week SC	Flu-like symptoms, injection site reactions, allergy, elevated liver enzymes, depression	32% reduction in ARR for high dose
Interferon beta-1b	Reduces BBB disruption and modulates T-cell, B-cell, and cytokine functions	250 μg on alternate days SC	Flu-like symptoms, injection site reactions, allergy, elevated liver enzymes, depression	34% reduction in ARR
Pegylated interferon beta-1a	Improved pharmacokinetic properties due to addition of PEG, mechanism same	125 μg once in 2 weeks SC	Injection site reactions, flu-like symptoms, fever, headache, infections	35% reduction in ARR
Glatiramer acetate	Competes with myelin basic protein to induce T-cell tolerance and stimulates regulatory T-cells	Low dose: 20 mg once daily SC; High dose: 40 mg thrice a week SC	Injection-site reactions, lipoatrophy, self-limiting episodes of flushing, chest tightness, dyspnea, palpitations, and anxiety during injection	29–34% reduction in ARR
Dimethyl fumarate	Activates nuclear factor E2-related factor-2 pathway which prevents neuronal death and myelin damage	240 mg twice a day orally	Gastrointestinal problems, facial flushing, leukopenia, rare cases of PML	53% reduction in ARR
Teriflunomide	Reduces activity of mitochondrial dihydroorotate dehydrogenase enzyme essential for pyramidine synthesis	7 mg or 14 mg once a day orally	Diarrhea, nausea, elevated liver enzymes, teratogenicity	31% reduction in ARR

Continued

Immunotherapy

Continued

Agent	Mechanism of action	Dose and route	Side effects	Remarks
Fingolimod	Sphingosine-1-phosphate inhibitor, traps lymphocytes in periphery	0.5 mg/day orally	Bradycardia, conduction block, macular edema, elevated liver enzymes, lymphocytopenia, hypertension, herpes virus infection	54% reduction in ARR. Needs monitoring at initiation of therapy for heart block
Natalizumab	Antibody to α4 subunit of integrins, prevents migration of lymphocytes to CNS	300 mg once in 4 weeks IV infusion	Headache, fatigue, arthralgia, anaphylactic reactions, PML	68% reduction in ARR
Alemtuzumab	Anti-CD52, depletes T, B and natural killer subtypes	12 mg/day IV for 5 days in first year; 12 mg/day IV for 3 days after 12 months	Infusion-associated reactions, infections, thyroid disorders, autoimmune disorders, agranulocytosis, fatigue, headache, rash	55% reduction in relapse rate #
Daclizumab	Interleukin 2 receptor modulator, decreases T-cell proliferation	150 mg every 4 weeks SC	Nasopharyngitis, upper respiratory infection, injection site pain, hepatic dysfunction, cutaneous reactions	54% reduction in ARR
Ocrelizumab	Depletion of CD20+ B-cells	600 mg every 6 months IV infusion	Infusion reaction, infections	46% reduction in ARR #. Approved for treatment of primary progressive MS
Mitoxantrone	DNA topoisomerase II inhibitor	12 mg/m² every 3 months IV infusion	Bone marrow suppression, cardiomyopathy, leukemia, infections	42% reduction in ARR. Approved for secondary progressive MS

ARR, annualized relapse rate; BBB, blood–brain barrier; CD, cluster of differentiation; CNS, central nervous system; DNA, deoxyribonucleic acid; IM, intramuscular; IV, intravenous; PEG, polyethylene glycol; PML, progressive multifocal leukoencephalopathy; MS, multiple sclerosis; SC, subcutaneous.

Note: All ARR compared to placebo except # compared to 44 μg SC interferon beta-1a.

CONCLUSION

With the better understanding of the immune system and advancements in molecular biology, the basket of immunotherapeutic drugs is ever expanding. These drugs are double-edged swords as they usher in risk of opportunistic infections and other rare adverse effects. Most of the drugs need prolonged and sometimes lifelong administration, which calls for the development of more specific and safer drugs.

TAKE HOME MESSAGES

- The treatment of autoimmune neurological diseases involves two phases—(1) treatment of acute relapses, and (2) long-term therapy to maintain disease remission
- Corticosteroids are the most widely used therapy for neuroimmune disorders and are effective in most of the diseases (GBS and multifocal motor neuropathy being notable exceptions), but chronic use is limited due to their numerous side effects
- Intravenous immunoglobulin and therapeutic PE have contrasting mechanism of actions, but are highly effective in acute therapy, especially in antibody-mediated disorders
- Long-term maintenance is achieved with oral steroids with or without a combination with cytotoxic therapy
- Among the newer immunomodulatory agents, the CD20 specific monoclonal antibody rituximab is probably effective in a wide spectrum of diseases.

SUGGESTED READINGS

1. Aksamit A. Neurosarcoidosis. Continuum Lifelong Learning in Neurology. 2008;14:181-96.
2. Allison AC, Eugui EM. Mycophenolate mofetil and its mechanisms of action. Immunopharmacology. 2000;47:85-118.
3. Amato AA, Greenberg SA. Inflammatory myopathies. Continuum (Minneap Minn). 2013;19:1615-33.
4. Atkins HL, Freedman MS. Hematopoietic stem cell therapy for multiple sclerosis: Top 10 lessons learned. Neurotherapeutics. 2013;10:68-76.
5. Bascić-Kes V, Kes P, Zavoreo I, et al. Guidelines for the use of intravenous immunoglobulin in the treatment of neurologic diseases. Acta Clin Croat. 2012;51:673-83.
6. Bello AE, Perkins EL, Jay R, et al. Recommendations for optimizing methotrexate treatment for patients with rheumatoid arthritis. Access Rheumatol. 2017;9:67-79.
7. Berkovich R. Treatment of acute relapses in multiple sclerosis. Neurotherapeutics. 2013;10:97-105.
8. Calabresi PA, Kieseier BC, Arnold DL, et al. Pegylated interferon β-1a for relapsing-remitting multiple sclerosis (ADVANCE): A randomised, phase 3, double-blind study. Lancet Neurol. 2014;13:657-65.
9. Chan ESL, Cronstein BN. Molecular action of methotrexate in inflammatory disease. Arthritis Res. 2002;4:266-73.
10. Chelbi-Alix MK, Wietzerbin J. Interferon, a growing cytokine family: 50 years of interferon research. Biochimie. 2007;89:713-8.
11. Chrousos G, Kattah J, Beck R, et al. Side effects of glucocorticoid treatment. Experience of the Optic Neuritis Treatment Trial. JAMA. 1993;269:2110-2.
12. Cortese I, Chaudhry V, So YT, et al. Evidence-based guideline update: Plasmapheresis in neurologic disorders: Report of the Therapeutics and Technology Assessment Subcommittee of the American Academy of Neurology. Neurology. 2011;76:294-300.
13. Costanzi C, Matiello M, Lucchinetti CF, et al. Azathioprine: Tolerability, efficacy, and predictors of benefit in neuromyelitis optica. Neurology. 2011;77:659-66.
14. Dalakas MC. B-cells as therapeutic targets in autoimmune neurological disorders. Nat Clin Pract Neurol. 2008;4:557-67.
15. Dalmau J, Lancaster E, Martinez-Hernandez E, et al. Clinical experience and laboratory investigations in patients with anti-NMDAR encephalitis. Lancet Neurol. 2011;10:63-74.

16. English C, Aloi JJ. New FDA-approved disease-modifying therapies for multiple sclerosis. Clin Ther. 2015;37:691-715.
17. Gold R, Dalakas MC, Toyka KV. Immunotherapy in autoimmune neuromuscular disorders. Lancet Neurol. 2003;2:22-32.
18. Gold R, Giovannoni G, Selmaj K, et al. Daclizumab high-yield process in relapsing-remitting multiple sclerosis (SELECT): A randomised, double-blind, placebo-controlled trial. Lancet. 2013;381:2167-75.
19. Goodin DS, Cohen BA, O'Connor P, et al. Assessment: The use of natalizumab (Tysabri) for the treatment of multiple sclerosis (an evidence-based review). Report of the Therapeutics and Technology Assessment Subcommittee of the American Academy of Neurology. Neurology. 2008;71:766-73.
20. Gorson KC, Amato A, Ropper A. Efficacy of mycophenolate mofetil in patients with chronic immune demyelinating polyneuropathy. Neurology. 2004;63:715-7.
21. Graves D, Vernino S. Immunotherapies in neurologic disorders. Med Clin N Am. 2012;96:497-523.
22. Hauser SL, Bar-Or A, Comi G, et al. Ocrelizumab versus interferon beta-1a in relapsing multiple sclerosis. N Engl J Med. 2017;376:221-34.
23. Killestein J, Rudick RA, Polman CH. Oral treatment for multiple sclerosis. Lancet Neurol. 2011;10:1026-34.
24. Kimbrough DJ, Fujihara K, Jacob A, et al. Treatment of neuromyelitis optica: Review and recommendations. Mult Scler Relat Disord. 2012;1:180-7.
25. Kitley J, Elsone L, George J, et al. Methotrexate is an alternative to azathioprine in neuromyelitis optica spectrum disorders with aquaporin-4 antibodies. J Neurol Neurosurg Psychiatry. 2013;84:918-21.
26. Kosmidis ML, Dalakas MC. Practical considerations on the use of rituximab in autoimmune neurological disorders. Ther Adv Neurol Disord. 2010;3:93-105.
27. Lallana EC, Fadul CE. Toxicities of immunosuppressive treatment of autoimmune neurologic diseases. Curr Neuropharmacol. 2011;9:468-77.
28. Lan N, Nguyen T, Cathala G, et al. Molecular mechanisms of glucocorticoid hormone action. J Mol Cell Cardiol. 1982;14 Suppl 3:43-8.
29. Markowitz CE. Interferon-beta: Mechanism of action and dosing issues. Neurology. 2007;68:S8-11.
30. Marriott JJ, Miyasaki JM, Gronseth G, et al. Evidence Report: The efficacy and safety of mitoxantrone (Novantrone) in the treatment of multiple sclerosis: Report of the Therapeutics and Technology Assessment Subcommittee of the American Academy of Neurology. Neurology. 2010;74:1463-70.
31. Martinelli, Boneschi F, Vacchi L, et al. Mitoxantrone for multiple sclerosis. Cochrane Database Syst Rev. 2013;5:CD002127.
32. Matsuda S, Koyasu S. Mechanisms of action of cyclosporine. Immunopharmacology. 2000;47:119-25.
33. Meriggioli MN, Ciafaloni E, Al-Hayk K, et al. Mycophenolate mofetil for myasthenia gravis: An analysis of efficacy, safety, and tolerability. Neurology. 2003;61:1438-40.
34. Morgenthaler JJ, Nydegger UE. Synthesis, distribution and catabolism of human plasma proteins in plasma exchange. Int J Artif Organs. 1984;7:27-34.
35. Mukhtyar C, Guillevin L, Cid MC, et al. EULAR recommendations for the management of primary small and medium vessel vasculitis. Ann Rheum Dis. 2009;68:310-7.
36. Novak JC, Lovett-Racke AE, Racke MK. Monoclonal antibody therapies and neurologic disorders. Arch Neurol. 2008;65:1162-5.
37. Patil US, Jaydeokar AV, Bandawane DD. Immunomodulators: A pharmacological review. Int J Pharm Pharm Sci. 2012;4 Suppl 1:30-6.
38. Patwa HS, Chaudhry V, Katzberg H, et al. Evidence-based guideline: Intravenous immunoglobulin in the treatment of neuromuscular disorders: Report of the Therapeutics and Technology Assessment Subcommittee of the American Academy of Neurology. Neurology. 2012;78:1009-15.
39. Randall KL. Rituximab in autoimmune diseases. Aust Prescr. 2016;39:131-4.
40. Ransohoff RM. Natalizumab for multiple sclerosis. N Engl J Med. 2007;356:26229.
41. Sanders DB, Wolfe GI, Benatar M, et al. International consensus guidance for management of myasthenia gravis. Neurology. 2016;87:419-25.
42. Sellner J, Boggild M, Clanet M, et al. EFNS guidelines on diagnosis and management of neuromyelitis optica. Eur J Neurol. 2010;17:1019-32.
43. Tenembaum S, Chamoles N, Fejerman N. Acute disseminated encephalomyelitis. A long-term follow-up study of 84 pediatric patients. Neurology. 2002;59:1224-31.
44. Thornton CA, Griggs RC. Plasma exchange and intravenous immunoglobulin treatment of neuromuscular disease. Ann Neurol. 1994;35:260-8.

45. Trebst C, Jarius S, Berthele A, et al. Update on the diagnosis and treatment of neuromyelitis optica: Recommendations of the Neuromyelitis Optica Study Group (NEMOS). J Neurol. 2014;261:1-16.
46. Van den Bergh PYK, Hadden RDM, Bouche P, et al. European Federation of Neurological Societies/Peripheral Nerve Society Guideline on management of chronic inflammatory demyelinating polyradiculoneuropathy: Report of a joint task force of the European Federation of Neurological Societies and the Peripheral Nerve Society - First Revision. Eur J Neurol. 2010;17:356-63.
47. van den Borne BE, Landewé RB, Goei The HS, et al. Cyclosporin A therapy in rheumatoid arthritis: Only strict application of the guidelines for safe use can prevent irreversible renal function loss. Rheumatology (Oxford). 1999;38:254-9.
48. Vermersch P, Stojkovic T, de Seze J. Mycophenolate mofetil and neurological diseases. Lupus. 2005;14:s42-5.
49. Vollmer T, Stewart T, Baxter N. Mitoxantrone and cytotoxic drugs' mechanisms of action. Neurology. 2010;74:S41-6.
50. Vurdelja RB, Friedrich L. Pulse glucocorticoid therapy in neuroimmune disorders. Neurol Croat. 2013;62:49-55.
51. Wingerchuk DM, Carter JL. Multiple sclerosis: Current and emerging disease-modifying therapies and treatment strategies. Mayo Clin Proc. 2014;89:225-40.
52. Winters JL. Plasma exchange: Concepts, mechanisms, and an overview of the American Society for Apheresis guidelines. Hematology Am Soc Hematol Educ Program. 2012; Plasma exchange: concepts, mechanisms, and an overview of the American Society for Apheresis guidelines. Hematology Am Soc Hematol Educ Program. 2012;2012:7-12.
53. Wood L, Jacobs P. The effect of serial therapeutic plasmapheresis on platelet count, coagulation factors, plasma immunoglobulin, and complement levels. J Clin Apheresis. 1986;3:124-8.
54. Zivkovic S. Intravenous immunoglobulin in the treatment of neurologic disorders. Acta Neurol Scand. 2016;133:84-96.